Lucy

The Anguish of Schizophrenia

SARAH W. HOLLOWAY

The names of some of the persons in this book have been changed or omitted in order to protect their privacy or to prevent embarrassment to them or to their families.

Library of Congress Control Number: 2008926175

LUCY: The Anguish of Schizophrenia *first published in 2008.*
Cover and Interior Designed by Amanda Butler, © 2008 Cold Tree Press
Cover Photographs of Lucy and Sarah by Expressions in Photography, Cookeville, TN
Cover Photograph, Illustration © iStockphoto.com / Hasan Kursad Ergan, Mark Stay

Printed in the United States of America
ISBN-13: 978-1-58385-263-7
ISBN-10: 1-58385-263-8

I Love You Friend

I love you friend
More than from the start of the salty ocean
To where it ends
More than the length and breadth of the great green prairies
Or the long stretching sandy shorelines
That penetrate the world's countries
The love I feel for you
Is full of such keen emotional warmth and caring
Compassion and sharing
That I cannot describe it
Except that it's a love
Whose depth is more than you can comprehend
My sweet, beautiful friend!

Lucy S Holloway

Lucy's Poem to an Unknown Friend, 1970s

INTRODUCTION

Much of this book was published as *What Happened To Lucy, A Story of Struggle in the Enveloping Tentacles of Schizophrenia,* copyright 1989. In the sixteen years that have passed since I wrote that book, so many things have happened to Lucy that I felt the need to revise and update her story. I wish I could write that tremendous progress has been made in the care, treatment, and understanding of the severe and persistently mentally ill (SPMI), but that is not the case. I hope this book will heighten public awareness of the suffering and needs of thousands of victims of this incurable brain disease.

Near the beginning of her seventeenth summer, in June of 1978, an illness called schizophrenia swept full-blown into our only daughter's life. For years, none of us realized what was happening to her and to us.

Since that alarming spring day in 1978, mental illness has become my middle name. Schizophrenia is a part of our family forever. I don't know if there are any words that can make plain what that means. I've tried to find some, for Lucy, and for all those patients and families whose suffering I share.

I have only my memories and journals to guide me in putting together this account of Lucy's twenty-seven years. At best, we see each other "through a glass darkly"[1] on this earth. Schizophrenia is an illness of darkness and distortion, a riddle of the brain that remains unanswered.

Schizophrenia is characterized by a regular smorgasbord of symptoms: withdrawal, bizarre behavior (speaking and acting in strange ways that nobody understands, hearing things that nobody else can, seeing things that nobody else does), emotions that change so rapidly the person is in tears one minute and laughing riotously the next. It's having "flat emotions," meaning no high or low feelings of any kind. It is not a split personality. As one author put it, a schizophrenic person can't get one personality together, let alone two or three.

As a mother, I'm the one who has a split personality. Part of me tries to function at a distance from the ever-present effect schizophrenia has on our family. Another part of me is locked into every frightening, frustrating struggle that has confronted Lucy in the past ten years.

It's as if Lucy has gone down the street and turned a corner into some cluttered, hazy alley. We can't see her clearly anymore. We catch glimpses, and sometimes she runs back and hugs us and laughs and talks about old, familiar things, and it's almost like she's back again. But then she's off once more, and all we have left is a shadow, and all we can hear are the hollow echoes of what used to be.

With every recurring bout of illness (psychotic break with reality and subsequent hospitalization), Lucy moved further from us until we could no longer talk to her as if she were one of us. She has become "one of them," a chronic mental patient.

At twenty-seven she has already suffered the consequences of being a mental patient in our society: stigma, discrimination, ridicule, the inability to get or keep a job, being avoided by others. Finally, she has been shut off completely from our world in the locked ward of a state mental hospital.

When did she cross that line from "us" to "them"? It's very hard to tell when that precious baby, lovable little girl or boy, enigmatic teenager, starts to become somebody different, somebody really strange.

This slow, sad realization is almost impossible to accept. It hurts, and I wonder who hurts the most, the victim or the rest of the family? I used to think it was me, the suffering mother, until I saw the fear and confusion in our daughter's lucid eyes, the avoiding, sidelong glances, maybe because she couldn't bear to see reflected on my face, no matter what kind of lopsided smile was pasted there, the reality that something horrible had happened to her and it wasn't going away. Yes, Virginia, there really is schizophrenia and manic depression, and nobody knows the cause and nobody has the cure.

In his book *Surviving Schizophrenia, A Family Manual*, Dr. E. Fuller Torrey speaks of schizophrenics as "the lepers of the twentieth century."[2] Schizophrenia, like leprosy, is a cruel and alienating illness. Its victims are slowly and inexorably cut off from the things all human souls cherish most: the ability to contribute through gainful work and the use of their talents to the society in which they live. Schizophrenia robs them of their sense of place in a world into which they can never fit.

This illness, now recognized as a brain disease, attacks people in their early teens and twenties, those fragile, blossoming years when they are still fumbling for their identities in a presently harsh, hectic, highly technical world. It scrambles their responses. Lucy seemed like someone being constantly thrown off balance, trying sometimes desperately to catch up, to be part of it all, the laughter and quick jokes of her peers, the easy accomplishments of youth. She never quite made it.

Now, we don't know who she is. How much is real and how much is the craziness we often see and hear? What would she be like if this hadn't happened? We can never know.

She used to have neat, vertical handwriting and a mind that worked like everyone else's. At least, we thought so then.

The world of mental illness is a world of endless questions and few answers. It's knocking on strange doors, grasping at books, conversations, and anything hopeful from a psychiatrist's mouth. It's reaching for enlightenment and finding mostly blank walls of darkness. It's feeling all the time that things will get better, that life will be normal again, but it never is. Lucy's mind went into a tailspin, and for her, it seemed to be all downhill.

Severe mental illness is the continuing death of dreams. For us, it was witnessing the death of Lucy's dreams and experiencing the death of ours for her. Most dreams die hard, but delusional ones are especially tenacious. They are all that's left to a mind gone astray.

Today, Lucy's room at home is filled with the fragments of those failed dreams: abandoned notebooks; college course books; books of inspiration, of quotations, of self-help guides with underlined passages—mute reminders of her battle to turn back the tide of confusion. For Lucy, nothing stemmed that tide except the drugs, and even they could not hold back the recurring onslaughts of illness.

I look at her almost empty "hope" chest, her Christmas gift on a day we never dreamed of sickness, and I grieve for those blocks of her life that schizophrenia has amputated. I remember her expectations, and ours, of marriage and motherhood, or of a career as a nurse, home economics teacher, psychologist, or nurse's aide. Eventually we just hoped for any kind of job that she might be able to do. Then we just hoped she could have some kind of a life outside of a hospital. I grieve because I didn't understand for so long what she was up against from the day of her first breakdown—a ruthless, relentless disease that was worse than anything I could imagine.

I remember going to the county library during those months after Lucy's first breakdown in search of more information about schizophrenia. The small collection of dated books there (most were twenty or thirty years old) were mainly technical, unintelligible psychiatric studies full of professional jargon and statistics, all numbingly depressing. Until Dr. Torrey's *Surviving Schizophrenia* was published in 1983, there seemed to be no book that gave families current information about schizophrenia that the average person could understand. It has become almost a bible among family support groups. Today there are a number of others available and more being written every day.

In Proverbs 18:14 it is written, "The spirit of a man will sustain his infirmity, but a wounded spirit who can bear?"[3] The chronically mentally ill are wounded spirits to a degree that most people cannot imagine. Their talents and abilities and dreams have long ago been lost in the continuing series of catastrophic breakdowns and hospitalizations and in the long years of trying and failing to "get well" so that they can function in the normal world again. Each failure to get better (to be normal) adds to the initial wounding—the destructive, shattering break with reality. The deep, unending loneliness that can result from all of this is terrible.

Our relationships to other people are what give life its meaning above all else. Severely mentally ill patients find it hard to relate to other people and sometimes even to pets. Lucy told me during the early years of her illness, "I don't know how to talk to anybody. There's a barrier between me and other people."

Communication isn't always easy in the normal world. We often see each other across chilly chasms of misunderstanding. But we have our bridges: shared love, laughter, tears, occupations, hobbies, and pursuits that bring us joy, satisfaction, and a sense of belonging. Lucy tries so hard to reach out when we visit. Her hugs, smiles, and effusive declarations of affection seem like desperate attempts to bridge an unbridgeable gap.

This alienation is one of the most painful aspects of schizophrenia. In those flashes of lucidity that come, we sometimes catch a glimpse of such sadness in our daughter's face that we are happy when she is babbling to her voices again, completely lost in another world. It's so much better than what may be her terrible awareness of what she, and we, have lost.

Whenever I awaken from a frightening dream at three o'clock in the morning and thankfully realize it was only a dream, I think of Lucy and how it may be for her. I hear someone on the staff at the state hospital saying, "She was crying and screaming some last night, but she's better today. She's pretty quiet this morning." I wonder if Lucy wakes in the night from terrible dreams, but the dreams are still there—the crazy, mixed-up, terrifying dreams—and the voices from the dreams are still talking to her, and no matter how much she cries or screams or what medicine she takes, they don't go away.

I hear Lucy telling my husband in a quiet, normal tone of voice as we sit in the spring sunshine under the trees at the state hospital, "Dad, why don't you put me to sleep? My head is all messed up—I don't want to live." I think of Lucy trying to talk to us, saying over and over, "I want to talk to you guys. I want to have a long talk with you, Mom," as she holds us both tightly. But the next instant she's talking to her voices, and she begins to yell at them louder and louder, and I lie in bed and cry because I can't do anything to change it.

This book tells a part of what has happened to Lucy. I have pieced it together as Lucy pieced her quilt during her last year at our farm, her last "real" days at home. It is pieced with bits from old scrapbooks, notes, journals, and memories etched in shock that have stayed in my mind when much else has faded. It isn't really Lucy's story—only she could tell that—anymore than the quilt she made is the old dresses, coats, and suits it's made of. It's only parts, some bright colors, some bits of yarn. Lucy's fragmented personality is like that for me.

I hope that what I've written will help Lucy understand what we have slowly come to believe—that nobody is to blame for mental illness. I hope it will give her some sense of her life as a whole and how much that life means to us, her family.

Many of the experiences in these pages will seem all too familiar to the millions of families who have a relative caught in the encircling darkness of schizophrenia. If this book helps in any way to bring more enlightenment to others, I will be, in Lucy's words, "well blessed."

In the ten years that have passed since the nightmare day when I first feared our daughter would be locked away, we have come to that still-not-fully accepted reality. She is locked away, physically and mentally. I remember asking a nurse on that first strange visit to the mental health center, "We haven't lost her, have we?"

She answered with a reassuring smile, "Oh, no. She'll be all right. You haven't lost her."

But we have lost her. The daughter that I could laugh with and fight with, cook with and cry with, share books and dreams and everyday life with, is lost; and I mourn and miss that loss every day of my life.

Lucy

Chapter One
OCTOBER 1982

"Please Don't Do This!"

Tuesday, October 5, 1982. My journal notes for that day begin, "One of the saddest days of our lives." It was mild and bright, an Indian-summer sort of day. Our small, two-story farmhouse and ten acres of woods and pasture looked peaceful. The red and gold leaves of several tall maples and walnuts near the house colored our ridge in a warm, autumnal glow, but the events of that day totally belied the tranquil, mid-afternoon milieu outside.

It had all started earlier that morning when Lucy, our twenty-one-year-old daughter, cheerfully kept an appointment with her psychiatrist at Plateau Mental Health Center, a voluntary treatment facility for those with mental problems in our section of Tennessee. Lucy was working on a cloth Humpty Dumpty doll at the time, and she took it along to show to her physician. We hoped she would sign herself in for treatment that morning. Her doctor had told us over the phone earlier in the week that if she didn't, he would probably have to have her committed to the state mental hospital in Chattanooga. "I believe she'll sign in, Mrs. Holloway," Dr. Johnson had told me over the phone. "Lucy has always been pretty good about taking my advice." I was praying that he was right.

My husband, Frank, and I knew that Lucy had been lying to us daily about taking her medicine, the vital element in controlling her illness, schizophrenia. We were sure that she was hardly ingesting any of it. Frank had been putting the medicine in orange juice, but we knew Lucy would soon catch on to this and refuse the juice. Our only hope of getting her the help we knew she needed was for her to sign in for treatment at Plateau that day.

This faint hope vanished when Frank drove home after the appointment and I saw Lucy in the front seat. We were now faced with something—forced commitment—that we dreaded and knew almost nothing about. Nobody at Plateau had explained how such things were handled, and my heart sank at the prospect.

It all seemed so unreal. Our gentle, shy daughter had become as frightening to us that week as a stranger in a scary movie. She had stayed in her room for days, talking to herself, laughing, switching her light on and off, and playing with an electric calculator she called her boyfriend. She talked to it constantly, chanting questions like, "If this is right, give me a number," and other comments that made no sense to us.

Turning the light on and off was a big part of this game, and her carpet bore the imprint of the seemingly endless trips she had made from her bed to the switch on the wall. I remember standing outdoors in the cool, autumn dusk, looking at her little upstairs window and watching that light go on and off, on and off, with a sickening, deepening dread.

For weeks, Lucy's behavior had been growing more strange and unpredictable. One frightening ritual she had started during this period had to do with the keys to our car. Every night she demanded that they be left on the fireplace mantel in a designated spot. Her father tried to bluff her out of this. We tried ignoring her directive. She became someone we didn't know, screaming and cursing in raging tones that stunned and amazed us. We left the keys on the mantel so we could get her to go upstairs to bed. Later, Frank would get them and keep them in our bedroom. The thought that she might slip downstairs and drive off into the night was a constant fear.

I felt only despair when I saw Frank and Lucy getting out of our car that morning. "Everything went fine," Lucy told me as they came inside. She was in good spirits but Frank looked drained. After Lucy had gone upstairs, we walked outside and he told me what had happened.

Frank had waited while Lucy kept her 10:30 appointment. After only a short time, Dr. Johnson called Frank into his office and asked Lucy to wait outside.

"Lucy's not going to sign herself in, Dr. Holloway, and there's no question about her needing to be hospitalized right now. I'm writing an emergency commitment order to Moccasin Bend Mental Health Institute (the nearest state hospital). I don't think there's anything more we can do here."

In the midst of this conversation, Lucy suddenly strode back into the room and demanded, "What are you doing?"

"I'm doing what I told you I was going to do, Lucy," Dr. Johnson replied.

Lucy reached forward, ripped the piece of paper from the doctor's hands, tore it into shreds, and informed him loudly, "I'm not going to any mental hospital. I don't need to be in a mental institution—you do."

Lucy's relationship with Dr. Johnson until that moment had been one of mutual respect. I think she looked on him as a fatherly figure of authority. She had told us once, "He reminds me of Uncle Bill." This act was unlike anything any of us could imagine her doing.

Dr. Johnson, calm and tightlipped, told Frank, "Just take her on home, and you come back."

Frank spent a good part of the rest of the day driving back to Plateau to pick up the commitment order and then waiting around the jail for hours for confirming telephone calls to be completed between the sheriff's office and Plateau Mental Health personnel. Nobody at either place seemed to understand or even be aware of his distress.

Lucy stayed in her room most of the afternoon, and I waited to hear something from Frank with growing anxiety. Finally, worn out from his ordeal, he drove home again and said wearily, "Two deputies are coming out in a little while."

My mind flew ahead toward finding some way of getting Lucy out of the house without a violent scene. I knew there was no way she would go willingly. Frank and I walked outside and stood waiting tensely on our porch, watching the front entrance drive some 500 feet down a sloping, graveled driveway.

After what seemed an eternity, we saw a car turn in. We met it as it pulled up near the house and spoke briefly to the two men who got out. The older one, big and stolid looking, listened without expression; the younger man seemed slightly apprehensive but sympathetic.

"We'll go in and bring Lucy out," I told them, searching their faces for understanding. I looked at Frank. "You go up and see if she'll come down." He nodded and went into the house while I stood beside the porch with the waiting men. I hoped Lucy hadn't seen the car approach.

Frank went upstairs to our blue-eyed daughter's room and knocked. "What is it?" she called, in a familiar, half-hostile, suspicious tone.

"Lucy, somebody outside wants to talk to you," Frank said, opening the door.

She was resting on the bed, her auburn-blonde hair slightly mussed. She looked at him blankly for a moment. "Okay," she said suddenly, getting quickly to her feet. After a cursory glance in the mirror and a few swipes at her hair with a brush, she followed him obediently out the front door into the October sunshine to see who waited for her there.

Everything happened quickly. Lucy's eyes widened in surprise as she saw the two uniformed men. Without comment, the officers took her firmly by the arms and began leading her to the marked patrol car with secured back seat cage. I don't remember what Lucy said in that awful instant, but her eyes met ours with shocked awareness of an unthinkable act. We followed, trying to explain to her why this desperate step had been taken, but her shrieks of protest, "Don't do this! Please! I'll take the medicine—I'll *take* the medicine now!" rang in our ears like hammer thuds.

We pursued the painful procession as they led her struggling figure inexorably toward the car. Her bare feet padding over the harsh, gray gravel and the short, royal blue, terry cloth exercise suit she'd been resting in, enhanced her defenselessness. She kept looking back at Frank and me in bewildered disbelief.

We had some notion the officers would talk with us as soon as Lucy was safely inside the automobile, but they got in the front seat and began moving abruptly away. We stared at the disappearing vehicle in stunned anguish, wondering what the journey of approximately one hundred miles to the state hospital would be like for Lucy.

"She doesn't have any clothes!" I said, snapping back to reality. "Why didn't they wait? She didn't even have on shoes! *Dammit!* Why didn't they *wait?*"

"Maybe we can stop them," Frank said. "I'll call the sheriff and see if he can't hold them up somewhere until we can get her clothes there."

We ran back into the house, and I dashed upstairs, grabbed Lucy's blue canvas overnight case from her closet, and began packing—

slippers, gown, duster, jeans, underwear, and a few other articles of clothing. I forgot toothbrush and comb in my haste and hurried downstairs to see what Frank had been able to do. "He's going to stop them at the jail until we get there," he said. "Let's go."

Churning with the accumulating anger, frustration, and grief of the past twenty-four hours, we drove the seven miles into town as fast as we dared on our mountain road. Ten minutes later we pulled up and parked next to the patrol car in front of the grim-looking jail.

The nightmare continued. Lucy's cries from the car's backseat brought quick tears to our eyes. "Please let me out. Please don't do this! I'll take the medicine now. Please!" The sight of her pleading figure crouched in the patrol car was bringing me to the brink of hysterical sobs.

A group of men just inside the jail offices looked on dispassionately. We transferred the bag of clothes to the drivers and asked them to give Lucy some slippers we'd brought in hand. Frank asked them to wait a minute.

"We can call Dr. Johnson and see if she can go to Plateau now," he said, turning to me. I nodded agreement, and we went inside and asked to use a telephone and for someone to tell the drivers to wait until we made the call. A man motioned us to a phone, and Dr. Johnson listened while I told him where we were and of Lucy's pleas and promises to sign in at the mental health center.

"Mrs. Holloway, I'm afraid it will all be to do over if you don't go through with it now," he said.

"Couldn't she just come out and talk with you again?" I asked. "She says she'll sign herself in now and that she'll take her medicine."

"I don't think it will do any good. I know it's hard, but sometimes people have been very thankful later that they took this step. There's really nothing more we can do here." His words rang with experienced finality. Frank and I went back outside to tell the officers.

We tried again to explain to Lucy why it was necessary for her to go to the state hospital, that Dr. Johnson thought it was the only way.

"No, no—you don't understand! I'll take the medicine now. Just let me out of here. Please, take me back to Plateau," she began again. The officers were ready to leave.

"We'll talk to her on the way." The younger deputy's voice broke through Lucy's shrill protests. "She'll be okay. She'll quiet down."

It was almost the first word either of them had spoken to us, and we turned to the younger man gratefully. "Yes, you will talk to her, won't you?" I asked.

Frank added in a ragged voice, "Just take care of her—take good care of her."

"Good-bye, Luce. We'll see you soon. We'll talk to you later." We spoke to her one last time through the window and watched in bleak silence as the patrol car swung out into the street and quickly disappeared.

It was almost six years later that we learned that one or both of us could have gone with Lucy in the patrol car that day. If we could not accompany her, a woman attendant was supposed to be with her. Apparently at that time, nobody at Plateau Mental Health Center or at the sheriff's office was familiar with 1984 Tennessee Code, Volume 6, 33-6-106: "Transportation of patient to hospital—Temporary detention," which states: "A female attendant shall always accompany a female patient to the hospital unless she is accompanied by one or more adult relatives."

Our daughter had been in and out of the local mental health center since 1978, but she had now embarked on a long, sad journey that would finally take her away from us almost completely. We didn't dream that she would never come home again to her sunny, yellow room with sloped ceilings at the top of the stairs.

We were four years into an enigmatic, destructive disorder of the mind—schizophrenia—that we still thought was going to get better.

"This illness doesn't tend to get better, Mrs. Holloway. It tends to get worse. The statistics aren't very encouraging in cases like your daughter..." What psychiatrist had said that to me? It didn't matter. I didn't believe it anyway. Depressing statistics were about other people, vague, shadowy souls locked away somewhere. Lucy would get better.

A red October sun was dropping behind the mountain ridges leaving a soft, vivid glow that touched the yellow and orange leaves of the fall-draped trees with an almost painful beauty. We drove home in the fading sunshine, seeing the road through a blur of exhausted tears.

“It’ll be dark soon,” I said numbly, imagining Lucy in the locked cage, moving along the winding road over the dark mountains, going toward strangers and unknown surroundings.

“She’ll be there in a couple of hours,” Frank said. “We’ll call the hospital.”

Chapter Two
MARCH 1961

"A Violet By A Mossy Stone"

Long ago I copied in the front of her pink baby book the second stanza of a poem by William Wordsworth. I thought the words were pretty and fitting for my beautiful baby daughter.

"Lucy
She dwelt among the untrodden ways…
…A violet by a mossy stone,
Half-hidden from the eye!
—Fair as a star, when only one
Is shining in the sky."[4]

In the past ten years Lucy has become more than half hidden from our eyes. Today we see only bits and pieces of the daughter we knew. It's as if she were serving a life sentence for a crime she didn't commit and doesn't understand. One of her continuing delusions is that she is in prison and is to be executed for "bad thoughts" or criminal acts that come to her mind out of the dark shadows of her illness.

Looking back, I can't remember anything being very easy for Lucy—not even getting born. It was March 1961. The details are hazy, but labor began late Tuesday morning. I went to the hospital with my husband after midnight, leaving my aunt with our two-year-old son, Frankie.

It was a wearing labor because she was not in the normal birth position and the doctor couldn't get her turned for delivery. After almost nine hours, I heard a nurse ask, "Aren't you going to give her anything?" I think he said something about having to take her with forceps. I was too tired to hear more. The next thing I remember, someone was saying, "You have a baby girl." They were happy words—enough to blot out everything else.

She arrived at 8:52 a.m. on Wednesday, March 22, 1961. She weighed in at nine pounds, four ounces, and had a cap of soft dark hair and blue eyes. I can still see the little indentations on either side of her forehead where the doctor had used the forceps. They gradually faded after the first week or two.

My mother told me later, "I kept calling the hospital until some snippy nurse in a sarcastic voice said, 'You must be the grandmother.' I told her, I *am* the grandmother, and I'm going to keep calling until I know my daughter and that baby are all right."

A nurse came in sometime later in the morning and said, "Your husband was really standing on his head for a while there."

I recalled these things because I was unused to being the center of attention in a hospital. At that time, I had never been in one except for the births of my children. I was thirty-three years old and having babies was the biggest adventure, the happiest and highest point of my life then. I talked about all of their births later, recalling in detail all the tiresome particulars of each one. Women love to tell childbirth tales—the grislier the better. I have heard since that one of the worst things a mother can do is to talk before children about the difficulties, if any, of their births, that it can be very disturbing to them later on. At the time, I never thought of it.

Years later, in the psychotic grip of her illness, sometime in the winter of 1981-82, Lucy accused me of hating her because her birth had been difficult. I don't know if I ever convinced her of the joy I felt that late March morning when she was born. I remember vividly the peaceful tiredness of a job well done when you can see your stomach isn't hiding your feet any longer and you know the baby has come and is all right.

I recall my happiness so clearly, especially when our pediatrician stopped by to say he had just examined her and answered with a twinkle my silent question.

"She's perfect," he said.

Chapter Three

JULY 1961 – FEBRUARY 1967

Earliest Days

What was she like, that plump, blue-eyed baby who had such a struggle getting into the world? Sweet, shy, affectionate, totally normal, and healthy. She slept on her tummy and loved being rocked. Like her brothers, she was breast-fed until weaned to a cup at about seven or eight months.

We brought her home from the hospital to a new, three-bedroom house in a beautiful, new subdivision in my hometown, Tallahassee, Florida. Frank was then working as a traffic engineer with the Florida State Road Department.

Frankie, almost two, was at first jarred by her arrival, but he soon found his way to love and acceptance of a baby sister and watched over her solicitously. He handed her toys in the playpen and soothed, "Don't pie, Looie," when tears erupted.

When she was about five months old, I wrote, "Lucy is wide awake and cheerfully sucking her thumb by 5:30 a.m. She looks up expectantly when I go in and rewards me with a joyful grin when I take her up."

In the spring of 1962, we moved to Cincinnati, Ohio, where

Frank had accepted a job as a consulting engineer in the heart of the city.

Lucy was a year old, very active, and almost brave enough to walk on her own. She started walking at about thirteen months and seemed delighted with her newfound ability. In May, I wrote, "Lucy is toddling about from room to room. She exhausts herself rushing around. Now she is pulling magazines and books off the coffee table. She is beginning to feed herself and talk some, saying, 'Hi!' with a lot of expression and a very fetching smile."

The months in Cincinnati were short. In July of 1962, my mother was ill, and we returned to Tallahassee where Frank took a job as a civil engineer with another consulting firm. We bought a beautiful, four-acre country home ten miles from town, and my mother, suffering from heart disease and other ailments of old age, came to live with us.

I had help for the first time, a black maid named Sarah who lived just through the woods from us. She loved the children and helped care for my mother, and we loved her. Frank mowed a path through the woods to Sarah's house so we could walk back and forth. It seemed an ideal existence. We had puppies, a cat, some chickens, and a fairyland of azaleas, dogwood, and camellias in landscaped gardens, a legacy from the former owner. I remember thinking that these must be my happiest years.

Lucy was almost three when Mark arrived on January 31, 1964. I'll never forget how forlorn she looked the day we brought him home.

"How is Lucy?" I kept asking Frank at the hospital. Children were not allowed to visit at that time, and I was worried about her reaction to my sudden absence. Frankie seemed to understand that I was in the hospital and would soon be home with a baby brother. Frank's report on Lucy—"She's been sort of sick with an upset stomach or something"—did nothing to allay my anxiety about her. Mark was a beautiful, healthy boy, and we were happy when we took him home on February 4. I could hardly wait to be with all the family again.

I remember going into the house through our garage that led into a big, yellow, country kitchen. I looked for Lucy at once. She was waiting with my mother as we came in. She was wearing a faded, slightly soiled, blue flannel nightgown I'd made for her, watching us silently with the most forsaken expression. I bent to hold her at once, but she was stiff and unresponsive. I felt like crying. I knew she must have thought I'd deserted her completely when I went to the hospital.

The following day I wrote, "Poor little Lucy felt bad, had fever, etc., while I was away, and I think she thought I had deserted her. She looked so unhappy when I got home yesterday; it broke my heart to see her, but is better today. She is pretty jealous of baby brother. Guess she can't understand why I can't lift her, etc. She doesn't like to see me rocking and nursing baby but hope she will get over this soon. She won't eat anything."

In her book *Necessary Losses,* Judith Viorst explains that we begin our lives with loss, cast from the womb and separated from our mothers, and she explains how painful this separation can be. She says this need for our mother's physical presence is absolute, and if we are separated before we are ready, before we can understand that the separation is only temporary, that our mother will return, the cost can be very high. Sometimes it can leave us forever fearful and uncertain, damaged, not fatally, but permanently.

One of my own earliest memories is fear of being parted from my mother, fear that she would leave me and never come back. That is why I felt so deeply the desolation I saw in Lucy's face the day we walked through the door with Mark.

Before Mark's arrival, Lucy and I took short naps together after lunch. She was cheerful and chatty, cuddling against me in the bed, and I wrote, "Lucy is so funny now. She loves to look at herself in the mirror and get dressed up in her 'Sunny School' dress."

After a few days of having a new baby, Lucy seemed better. She was soon kissing her baby brother, and all seemed normal until a trip we made to visit my half-sister, then in a nursing home in Selma, Alabama. One disturbing thing that I remember about that trip was Lucy's sudden, inexplicable silence. She withdrew from us totally and refused to speak, even to answer a question.

I made no notation of it in my journal at the time (so many things were happening that summer), but the memory is clear. I did mention it in later journal notes, and it worried me a lot. I fretted about it to Frank, who told me, "The more you carry on about it, the longer she's not going to talk." He thought I was making too much out of nothing and making it worse by worrying. Now, I sometimes wonder if this early withdrawal was an ominous symptom of the "slow insidious" approach of schizophrenia. All I knew then was that a strange, solemn silence had enveloped our sweet, talkative little girl, and I wanted her back.

Those childhood years went by so fast we had little time for reflection, but my journal for the summer and winter of 1964, has a number of entries about Lucy.

"Lucy very cross at times—cries a lot and appetite poor which worries me. She and Frankie fuss a lot—wish Frankie had some other boys to play with."

"Lucy cries at the drop of a 'no' these days. She races to the porch and flings herself into the swing where she awaits the sympathetic approach of someone before joining the family again."

"Lucy going to kindergarten with Frankie tomorrow to visit. Hope she will enjoy it. She is sleeping in room with Mama for past two nights, and being in with Grandma seems just what she needed. She is sleeping better and seems quite content about going to bed. It was really beginning to fray our nerves having to battle with her about bedtime and then be waked up during the night when she wanted to get in our bed. She's at a bad time I guess, with Frankie getting attention by going to kindergarten and Mark by being the 'baby,' she feels left out."

"Cool, rainy morning. Lucy is on porch, spreading blocks, cups, spoons, spools, etc., all over the floor and on sofa and carrying on a spirited conversation with herself. I just told her not to put any small objects out where Mark could get hold of them, and she responded,

'No. I ike him to get hold of them!' Very cooperative."

"Lucy is so excited about Santa, she forgot about not talking to us and talked and talked to her Daddy tonight."

"Lucy is asleep on the sofa—all worn out. She still doesn't talk very much. I really miss her chatter, but she goes silently about, dragging her dolls here and there, changing their clothes, feeding, bathing them, etc., and only occasionally breaks down and really talks to us. Try not to notice too much as afraid it will make her continue even longer."

A new year began but the problem with Lucy's silence continued, and I find this notation in January 1965: "Lucy is still having a difficult time for some reason. If I knew what troubled her, would try to correct it, but she has decided to continue life in silence so not much can do about it. Don't think she uttered a sound all day yesterday or today either. She is old enough to know we mean it when we tell her to do something, but she purposely ignores requests until she is spanked. Am really surprised when I tell her to do something and she does it. Usually have to force her to mind. One thing she does faithfully is help me when I change Mark by putting the soiled diaper in bucket. Surely hope her silence will not continue too long. Try to get her out and do all can to keep her happy but sometimes looks as if none of it helps."

In the summer of 1965, I noted, "Lucy still wants to be 'little' and says she's growing little, not big, when anybody says she's getting to be a big girl. Mark is her rival, but she and Frankie play together real well these days. Of course, they have fights but on the whole are quite companionable. Possibly this summer is last time they will play together in just this way as school will make a difference in Frankie and kindergarten in Lucy."

Lucy took her first long steps away from home in September 1965. She started kindergarten at Byrd-Wood School and attended from September 1965 until January 1967. She was only four, six months shy of the regular starting age, but we thought the contact with other children would help her shyness and an inability to communicate, which still persisted. Frankie had graduated from Byrd-Wood and started first grade, and she missed his company.

Lucy found her first real chum, Tammy, at Byrd-Wood kindergarten. I don't remember just when it was during the period from September to January 1967 that Tammy and her sister June became a part of our lives. We lived in the country; they lived right in town, and we visited back and forth regularly. Tammy's mother and I became friends and enjoyed being together while our children played. Lucy began looking forward to kindergarten because Tammy would be waiting for her every day. Tammy and June had a wonderful, almost-like-a-real-house playhouse in their backyard, which their father had built. Lucy especially loved playing there. Tammy was the opposite of Lucy—quick, confident, and outgoing—but they played together extremely well.

One of the teachers at Byrd-Wood told us sometime later that, while it was nice that Lucy and Tammy were friends, it was a one-sided friendship. Lucy was completely the follower and Tammy always the leader. I worried some about this, but I was so glad Lucy had a friend to play with; I didn't think it mattered too much.

Tammy and three other little girls from Byrd-Wood came to Lucy's first birthday party, her fifth, on March 22, 1966. Frank took movies of it, and the weather was perfect, a beautiful spring day in the country with blooming azaleas and camellias to match the bright dresses of the four little girls. They played in the small playhouse Frank had built on stilts in our back woods and ate ice cream and cake on the patio. Lucy seemed to enjoy it all, but her problem with communication was still there. It was hard for me to tell whether she was happy or not.

A note from Byrd-Wood's teachers, written May 30, 1966, seems to affirm our expectations about kindergarten helping Lucy. It reads: "Lucy has come a long way in overcoming her shyness and timidity this year. She is immature and still finds it hard to adjust to new situations very readily but tries hard and is making real progress. She does very nice handwork and has good eye-hand coordination, which is so necessary for writing, etc., later on. We're sure she will grow up a great deal this summer, and we're all looking forward to a happy year in kindergarten."

Frank and I were pleased with this note and also Byrd-Wood's report of that period, which indicated Lucy was able to get along with adults and other children, follow directions and routine, and show interest in and participate in all the activities. Overall, we were happy and unworried about her ability to adjust to school even though we knew it was difficult for her.

A disquieting note came with the next and last report from

Byrd-Wood, which read as follows: "Byrd-Wood Kindergarten, January 27, 1967, Dear Mr. and Mrs. Holloway: We know that you, as well as we, are aware of the progress Lucy has made the past year. At the same time, however, we feel that we should express to you our concern over her chances for happiness and success in the first grade next year. Lucy has a difficult time understanding directions and following them, and unless there is a good deal of growth between now and September, which, of course, is not impossible, we believe that she will be more mature and thus more able to cope with first grade work if she has another year in some good kindergarten.

"At this time Lucy's attention span is very short and she is easily distracted. When she has difficulties, she is very much disturbed. She is very shy, and, although we can encourage her to come up before the class with things she brings to share, she finds it too difficult to talk about them and can only hold them up for the class to see. We believe these difficulties are only the result of immaturity and that time and experience will take care of them.

"The above is only our opinion formed from years of experience with kindergarten and first grade children, but we are not experts. We would, therefore, like to urge you to take Lucy to a Human Development Clinic and be guided by their advice as to her readiness for more advanced work. Tragedy is sometimes the result of trying to force progress for which a child is not ready.

"We sincerely hope that you will take this letter in the spirit in which it is intended. We have all learned to love Lucy, and it is with regret that we are losing her. Sincerely..."

I was thankful for the interest and attention Lucy had received from her teachers at Byrd-Wood, but felt her immaturity would give way as she grew older. I reasoned, if she couldn't be a little immature in kindergarten, when could she be?

We were optimistic and full of plans that fall and winter. Frank had been looking into a teaching job at Louisiana State University in Baton Rouge, and made the decision to take it, which meant major changes in all of our lives.

The small worry I felt when I read the last letter from Lucy's kindergarten teachers soon vanished in a flurry of moving preparations.

Chapter Four

FEBRUARY 1967 – AUGUST 1974

The Growing Years

I remember our move to Baton Rouge, Louisiana, in February 1967, as a time of happy expectations, but also a time of tension and upheaval for our whole family. For Mark, two years old, it was his first move. For seven-year-old Frankie and five-year-old Lucy, it was their second uprooting and first parting from playmates they'd come to know well and depend on. For my mother, then eighty, it meant leaving my brother and his family and other relatives and friends in a town she'd lived in for forty-five years. For my husband, it was leaving a consulting job to enter a new field of teaching and study as Assistant Professor of Civil Engineering at Louisiana State University.

Our almost three years in Baton Rouge, from February 1967, to August 1969, began and ended with strain and loss. Frank's mother died of heart conditions in May 1967, our first spring in Louisiana. My mother died of congestive heart failure in July 1969, only a couple of weeks before we moved back to Tallahassee.

A thread of sadness will always run through my memories of that period. My mother's failing health and increasing feebleness, her breast cancer surgery in 1968, all the wearying trips to doctor's offices, and her last temporary stay in a nursing home dominated those years for me.

We started out with a spirit of adventure and high hopes in our rented house, which had a huge green lawn and shade trees. We enjoyed exploring the new stores and surroundings and the campus of Louisiana State University where Frank was teaching.

In April I wrote, "We're going to have Lucy checked over at Louisiana State University to test her readiness for first grade. She seems fine at times, then seems to have a lot of trouble communicating."

Lucy took a series of evaluation tests at the Human Development Clinic at LSU that June, and they thought she should go ahead to first grade, that holding her back, even though she was a little immature for her age, might be more detrimental.

We moved into our first custom-built house near campus in August 1967, and Lucy attended kindergarten at the school where she would be going to first grade in the fall. She seemed to enjoy it a lot and looked forward to regular school. Another journal note that summer reads: "Lucy has taught Mark all the songs she learned at kindergarten, and they loudly sing, 'Ring Around the Rosie,' 'Mary Had a Little Lamb,' and, loudest of all, 'Old McDonald Had a Farm.'"

Lucy and Frankie took private swimming lessons in July, and I wrote: "Lucy has really done well. I saw her swim yesterday and am thrilled at progress both of them have made."

As I remember those days now, I wonder what it was like for our three children when they were growing so fast and we were moving almost every three years. I know I was an energetic, omnipresent (I never worked away from home), and probably a domineering figure to all of them. I was indelibly marked by the wounds and conflicts of my own childhood. My earliest memories of life are partly happy (rocking before a fire in my mother's lap) and partly sad and fearful. I was afraid my mother would leave me, of shadows on the wall, bumps in the night, of being lost, ridiculed, and rejected. These are probably common fears for everyone, but I didn't know it then. I feel sure my fearful, over-imaginative nature colored my performance as a mother, but I remember my children's births and childhoods as some of the happiest years I've known.

I rocked them, played with them, and planned outings, birthday parties, and projects for them. Frank and I centered our lives around home and the children. We took camping trips and day trips to the state parks in Florida, Louisiana, Arkansas, and Mississippi. Our vacations were always spent on planned family trips. I loved camping—the smell of the big green and yellow canvas tent we bought in Baton Rouge, being away from regular routines, and the feeling of adventure.

I know I was often impatient and irritable. I look back and see a thousand things I wish I had done differently, but I try not to torture myself now for not being what I wanted so much to be then: a perfect wife, mother, sister, and daughter.

There were happy times for all of us in Baton Rouge, and a journal entry in March 1968 describes one of those almost-perfect days we sometimes forget to treasure at the time: "Yesterday was lovely all day. Frank took children to Sunday school. It was a beautiful, spring-like day. We went for a walk, then stayed home all day and watched children playing. Mama sat in the swing a little. I cut grass, sat in the garden, and thought how peaceful and happy a time it is just now for us. Can't help but wonder where all the children will be in ten years…

"Lucy took her Baby Secret doll out for some air and Frankie played with Hernandez (neighbor boy). Lucy is doing real good work at school. She reads a library book just about every day. She'll be seven on the 22nd—got to plan for a little party, Easter egg hunt, etc. Friday after next." I'm glad I couldn't see what was ahead for Lucy in ten short years on the shining spring day I wrote the above.

Frank's decision to work on his doctoral degree in the fall of 1968 changed our lives again. He had thought he could take a leave of absence from LSU, but this proved impossible, and by the spring of 1969, he was looking for another university to pursue his education.

The indecision about where and when we would move, coupled with my mother's worsening health, made our last months in Baton Rouge anything but tranquil. Finally, the decision was made. We would be moving back to Tallahassee where Frank would enter a program at Florida State University in August 1969. I was happy about going home and hoped my mother could live a few more years after we were settled. Her death in July was the lowest point of those last months of indecision and stress.

I returned to Tallahassee under a crushing load of grief and guilt. It seemed that everything that had ever bothered me in my life came stalking from the closets of my brain to drown me in a depression I couldn't pull out of. I relived every cross word I'd said to Mama during days of strain and frustration and couldn't forgive myself for the times I'd yelled hurtful things. I went to bed in tears, woke up in tears, and felt at any moment I might find myself unable to function at all.

A friend of my mother's suggested a psychiatrist, and for the first time I became familiar with a part of medicine that was to be a constant in our lives a few years down the road. I managed to carry on normally at home and I don't think the children were aware of my problems then. I spent about six months going to the psychiatrist for weekly psychotherapy, and the depression gradually lifted with the passage of time.

Mama had lived with us for seven years; her death was a loss for the children too. Frankie had reacted with tears when he saw his grandmother at the funeral home, and Mark was too young to show much emotion, but something about Lucy's reaction stayed in my mind. Whenever she saw me crying, she would start to smile. Lucy had shared a room with her grandmother, and I knew she loved her. I couldn't understand her seeming lack of grief, and her smile irritated me. I remember asking her sharply, "What's so funny, Lucy?"

She looked uncomfortable and answered, "I can't help it. I don't mean to laugh—I just can't help it. Don't *look* at me like that!"

I was to hear that admonition a lot in the future when I found it difficult to follow Lucy's pattern of thought. At the time, it worried me some, but I didn't attach any real significance to it. I don't know today if there was any. I regret confronting her in a scolding way for something she obviously couldn't help.

Our grief was made easier by the continuing demands of everyday life. Our first weeks in Tallahassee vanished quickly as we painted and refurbished our new home and investigated a nearby school where Frankie and Lucy would soon be going. We had nice neighbors and loved our house, which had a big, fenced backyard with shade trees for our dog, Gypsie, and a large, fruit-bearing fig tree just outside our back door.

Mark later enrolled in kindergarten at Hartsfield Elementary School, where Frank and Lucy were, and all three walked to and from school together.

Aside from my own personal conflicts and battle with depression, those years seemed to be happy, productive ones. Frank finished the course work for his doctorate, and the children appeared to be fairly comfortable with schools and friends, although, again, Lucy had no close chums. Her grades were mostly honor roll, and I don't recall any really upsetting events. I remember Lucy's fifth grade teacher telling me once, "Lucy will be fine if she doesn't get an ulcer before she's twenty."

This teacher took a special interest in helping Lucy and was concerned about her almost over-conscientious attention to her school work. "She's such a perfectionist," she told me, "But other than that, she's doing just fine."

I was glad to be in Tallahassee where I was born and was married, and where all of our children were born. We saw relatives and old friends and bought forty acres in an adjoining county. We planned to build a home there when Frank finished his doctoral work, and we spent a lot of time at our "place." Frank built a red barn storage house there where we kept chairs and other equipment. We hacked a trail down to a clear, sandy-bottomed little creek that ran through the back of the property and spent hours exploring the woods and fields.

All of us played badminton in our backyard. We installed a goldfish pool, and Frank built another storage barn there. Lucy did a lot of babysitting for our next-door neighbor who had a little girl about two years old. Years later, when we were living on a farm near Cookeville, Tennessee, Lucy still got letters from Marcie. She loved reading to the child and patiently entertained her for hours at the time. It made up for her lack of friends her own age during that time.

We became fairly active members of a nearby Methodist Church, and Lucy and Mark both sang in the choir at one time. We took day trips to the beaches near Tallahassee and camped near the Ochlockonee River and on the beaches of Panama City, St. Joseph Peninsula State Park, and St. Augustine. We took a memorable boat ride down the swift-flowing, tea-colored currents of the Suwannee River in the Stephen Foster Folk Culture Center State Park near Live Oak, and visited Marjorie Kinnan Rawlings's home in Cross

Creek, near Gainesville, where she wrote *The Yearling*. The trips and the years all run together, and through them all was a restless search for Frank and me and our separate desires. His was for a job that suited his training and disposition and mine was for a farm.

We had hoped to move to our forty acres near Tallahassee when Frank finished his work at Florida State, but he was unable to find a job in the area at that time. We put our home up for sale and prepared to move again in the summer of 1973. The only job Frank was able to find at the time was as a consultant in Miami, a place none of us had any desire to live.

"There aren't any trees in the yard," I said, when I told the children about the house in Dade County, which Frank and I had hastily settled on after a hurry-up trip to find a place before moving the family.

"Aren't there any trees at all?" Mark asked.

"Not a single large shrub," I assured him, thinking of the small, cramped yard that went with our house, which was in a nice subdivision in South Miami. We had chosen it because of its proximity to good schools and to Frank's work, the paramount considerations in that area.

We made the long, hot trip to Miami the last week in August. Lucy was suffering from ear and respiratory infections that made her first days in the new location miserable. I remember getting up in the night to give her aspirin for the awful headaches that kept her from sleeping.

Our new home was carpeted in shag, which had been liberally

sprinkled with tiny pebbles by neighborhood children while the house was under construction. It was also occupied by armies of ants and giant cockroaches that had established residence during the same period.

With the help of our next-door neighbor, we found a good doctor for Lucy, who needed immediate treatment for the infections; we vacuumed pebbles for weeks, and coped with a temporarily non-functioning air-conditioner, a year-round necessity in Miami.

Soon after moving in, we became acquainted with a large, friendly family down the street who had four daughters and one son living at home. One of the girls was Lucy's age, and these friends became our Miami "family" during the year we lived there. I think that year may have been one of the happiest for Lucy as I look back. She finally had someone to play with, ride bikes with, and walk or bike to school with. I believe she enjoyed that time more than she had any since she played with Tammy and June in their backyard playhouse in Tallahassee before our move to Louisiana.

All of us bicycled for miles along the flat, sunny thoroughfares. We dug holes in the coral rock, poured in peat and black dirt, and planted trees and shrubs around our small yard. We visited Miami's crowded beaches, the Everglades, and Key West, and spent a short vacation in Naples before our move to Cookeville, Tennessee.

Frank had to commute about eight miles through whizzing traffic every day, and he began looking for another job after six months in Dade County. We were more than happy to leave South Florida when he secured a position as Associate Professor of Civil

Engineering at Tennessee Tech University in Cookeville in the spring of 1974.

We stopped for a brief visit to Disney World on our hectic drive from Florida to Tennessee that August. We moved ourselves in a rented U-Haul truck, a packed station wagon, and a small trailer, and arrived in Cookeville during drenching rains after hours of tense driving. I vowed never to move again.

I knew that new schools and severed relationships with our friends in Miami would be hard, especially for the children. I still expected happy things and new adventures in Tennessee, which I had always thought was a beautiful state.

Lucy was thirteen that summer, Frankie was fifteen, and Mark was ten. All of us were healthy, and I was full of optimism about the future.

Chapter Five

AUGUST 1974 – JUNE 1978

"Something's Happened To Lucy!"

"This is the rainiest place I've ever seen," Frankie said gloomily in the midst of our unpacking activities in Cookeville that first week of August 1974.

"It's rained every day since we got here," echoed Lucy. The skies eventually cleared, and the weeks flew by as we learned the streets of our new town, put up a storage building in our backyard, cut the knee-high grass in our yard, and purchased the empty lot next door where we planned to have a big garden in the spring.

I was thrilled with the rural scenery, the beauty and size of Cookeville, the Tennessee Tech campus, and I was totally in love with Tennessee. I knew the hardest thing for all the children would soon begin—new schools. They would all be attending different ones. Frankie would be at Putnam County Senior High, Lucy at Cookeville Junior High, and Mark at Sycamore Elementary, which was just up the street from our house. September saw them all making the difficult transition of being new kids at strange schools again. It wasn't easy for any of them, but junior high was a real trial for Lucy.

We had become used to the easy, accepting atmosphere of Miami's polyglot population, and we missed the few friends we had gotten to know there. In Miami, nobody knew, and cared less, where you were from, who your ancestors were, and whether you did or didn't attend church. First-name friendships formed casually and quickly compared to our new town. Our immediate neighbors were friendly, and I thought school adjustments and friends would soon take care of themselves.

All of us had to get new eyeglasses that fall, and we discussed with the optometrist Lucy's problem with a slight walleye or "lazy eye" condition she had had for some time. He suggested eye exercises, which she did for several years.

Time passed quickly that fall and winter as we added an addition to our house, kept up with the children's school activities, and, in December, purchased ten acres in rural Putnam County to build our farmhouse. Lucy babysat for our neighbors, helped with yard work, cooking, and housecleaning, and made honor roll grades at school that year.

Frank and I gave Lucy a small cedar chest our first Christmas in Cookeville. I remember she polished it until it glowed. "This will make a good hope chest," I told her as we put away some special linen and a few other treasures, thinking of her future career or marriage.

In January 1975, Lucy began taking art lessons from a Lutheran minister's wife. She was a warm, attractive woman with a sweet, outgoing personality. She encouraged Lucy, and Lucy liked going to her house for the lessons. She still had no close friends, but she enjoyed the fellowship with some other students who had signed up for the course.

We took a camping trip to Fall Creek Falls State Resort Park in Tennessee in June 1975, just before we began construction of our farmhouse. I wrote, "It's the first time we've been camping in about three years. It may be the last one in a while that we all take together. Children are growing and so much togetherness no longer appealing." We enjoyed the park, but for Frankie and Lucy, camping as a family had lost much of its charm. This would be the last camp that all of us made together.

In the school picture she had made when she was fourteen, in the spring of 1975, Lucy wears a scooped-neck, blue and white print cotton dress that I had made for her and smiles into the camera. Her hair is parted in the middle, hanging in reddish brown waves as it falls to just below the shoulders, curling softly against the bodice of the dress. She had plucked her eyebrows to thin arches, but the eyes above the smiling mouth are almost blank. Studied separately, it's hard to find in them much humor or joy.

In a pencil drawing self-portrait she copied from this picture, she has captured the hair style, scooped-neck dress, and arched eyebrows, but the eyes are large and haunted looking, and the mouth is pinched and sad. There is a lost look about the picture. Another self-portrait, done on notebook paper with marker pencils in 1970, when she was nine years old, shows the same sadness of expression in mouth and eyes. Did she see herself more truly than we knew, even then?

During the early winter and spring of 1975, Lucy and I began attending a girls for Christ group that met at our church. It was later called Pioneer Girls, and a journal note in June reads, "Lucy baked brownies and delicious gingerbread for Pioneer Girls bake sale tomorrow."

During that same year, Lucy worked as a volunteer candy striper at Cookeville General Hospital, and we talked about her pursuit of a nursing career. That August I wrote, "Lucy likes her candy stripe work at the hospital. She got a book about candy stripers from the library yesterday."

One bright note from junior high came in January 1976. "Lucy got a part (Cynthia) in the play she wanted, and she has been studying her lines. Now she's making pancakes for Frankie and Mark."

The play took up Lucy's free time for the next several weeks, and in February, I wrote, "Lucy is immersed in her play, and if she misses any of her lines, I could probably understudy for her, have heard it so much!"

Reunion on Gallows Hill opened at Cookeville Junior High School the latter part of February for two performances and was a big success. Frank and I went and were very proud of Lucy's acting; she didn't miss a line. On February 28, I wrote, "Lucy went to Nashville with her play group to compete in performances at Belmont College today."

The play seemed to be the highlight of Lucy's last year at junior high. Her sophomore and junior years at Putnam County Senior

High weren't memorable for any particular events that I can recall or noted in my journal from that time. I know Lucy was often lonely, and I kept hoping she would get involved in some activity other than going to school and coming home day after day.

Lucy got her learner's permit and took some private driving lessons in the spring of 1977 when she was sixteen. Frank and I were not impressed with her instructor, a Tennessee Tech student, who often showed up late for the lessons. He was handsome and ingratiating to Lucy, however, and she proclaimed him "a wonderful teacher—he showed me how to drive on the interstate yesterday."

Lucy got her driver's license after a nervous, tension-filled morning (I went with her) at the Highway Patrol station. She practiced driving frequently after that, but she had an accident while driving with Frank in May. He had told her to slow down, but she panicked and hit the gas pedal instead. The station wagon door was damaged when they finally came to a shaky stop, but nobody was hurt. The incident shook our confidence in Lucy's ability to handle driving, and she didn't practice regularly after that. I didn't encourage her to keep at it and was relieved when she didn't mention wanting to drive. On New Year's Day 1978, I wrote, "Lucy wants to practice driving again—she still needs a lot before driving alone."

The winter of 1977-78 was severe. The children missed a lot of school because of the snow and icy roads, and I thought spring would never come. We celebrated Lucy's seventeenth birthday at home on March 22, 1978, with a steak dinner and a chocolate cake with white frosting. We sang "Happy Birthday" at the table while she opened her gifts: a record from Mark, then fourteen; a wallet from Frankie, then eighteen; and a little cross necklace she had wanted from Frank and me.

Lucy taught a Sunday school class for small children at our church that spring, and she spent a lot of time preparing for it. I worried about the extra burden of this class in addition to her schoolwork. With Lucy, there always seemed to be extremes. Either she wasn't doing enough (withdrawal) or she undertook what seemed to be too much. I didn't have confidence in her ability to handle a lot of things with balance. I'm sure she absorbed my lack of trust and that it wasn't helpful. I spoke to her about the Sunday school class a couple of times. "Lucy, you don't have to teach this class. Maybe you're trying to do too much."

"No, no. I love doing it," she always replied, and she seemed to enjoy planning for it each Sunday.

Frank and I had started building a farmhouse on our ten acres in June of 1975, and that spring and summer we were trying hard to finish it so we could move in. We were also trying to sell our house in town. Our whole family worked on the farmhouse at different times for about three years. Frank and I spent most of our free weekends and afternoons staining woodwork, painting, and seeing to the thousand and one details of getting the house completed. We were also sorting and packing our belongings in town. It was a period of hard work, and the days all tended to run together.

Lucy and I talked about a career for her in nursing during this period. "Maybe I could be a Red Cross worker," she said. I didn't know much about what was available and sent off for some material in the health services field for her.

My mother had been a nurse, a graduate of the University of Maryland, class of 1910. I admired the profession and had wanted to be a nurse myself. My first embroidery project, done when Lucy was a baby, was of a little girl in a nurse's uniform with cross-stitch lettering that read, "When I Grow Up."

I made a nurse's outfit for Lucy out of an old sheet when she was ten years old. She played with this costume a lot, and we got a doctor's play case with stethoscope, plastic thermometer, and bandages at the dime store and took her picture as a future nurse. I thought a career in nursing would be wonderful for Lucy, that it would give her the self-confidence and sense of identity she always seemed to lack. It was a dream career I fervently hoped might come to pass. Years later, during a bad period in her illness, Lucy broke up the framed, embroidered nurse and cut up the material.

I remember in late May, Lucy seemed to have a tremendous amount of energy. She helped me clean house. She took some long walks, at least four or five miles at a time. She made trips to the library and to restaurants where she applied for jobs. I recall my surprise when she came in the door from these outings and told me how far she had walked. "Good Heavens, Luce! Aren't you tired?" I asked.

"No, I enjoyed it. I got a little tired on the way home, but I'm fine," she answered.

Mark was in a play at junior high that spring. Frank and I went, but Lucy seemed preoccupied and didn't want to go. School was winding down, and we were absorbed with finishing the farmhouse and selling the house in town. I remember thinking how glad I would be that Lucy wouldn't have to ride the school bus anymore after we moved. Frank could drop her off on his way to the university.

Lucy's experiences on the school bus during our first years in Cookeville had horrified me. She would often come home crying and rush to her room. When I tried to find out what happened, she would sob something like, "Nobody would let me sit down. They put books on the seat, and nobody would let me sit by them!"

My heart ached for her pain, and I was angry too. Once she came home in a torrent of tears. I followed her to her room, finally coaxing from her what had happened. "Some boys spit on me out of the window when I got off," she said.

I was furious. I couldn't understand why anyone could or would want to treat anybody like that. I just couldn't imagine it happening to Lucy. I didn't know how to comfort her or what to tell her about how to handle it.

Lucy had applied for jobs at several fast-food restaurants, but none of them ever phoned for an interview. At the end of May we thought we had a sale for the house in town and were busy planning our move to the country. Frank had to make a trip to Atlanta in mid-June, and we had talked of working in a week's vacation trip to the beach. We thought Myrtle Beach, South Carolina, would be a nice break for the whole family as soon as school was out. Frankie had registered for summer classes at the university and was going to work at a convenience store.

I recall some vague anxiety about Lucy's sudden spurts of energy and a few "odd" remarks her brothers reported, but we were used to her being a little different. I never dreamed these might be symptoms of anything serious. I also worried about the sudden intensity of her religious ideas and the frequency and fierceness of family quarrels that seemed to spring up out of nowhere like black thunderclouds on sultry, summer afternoons. Lucy and I especially got into shouting, vindictive disputes that ended sullenly, incomplete and smoldering until the next flare-up. My conscious mind perhaps refuses to acknowledge real causes, but I can't remember what they were about now.

I know they were contests of will. I felt a desperate need to stay in control—I felt my authority as a mother was threatened and challenged, which is probably normal for most mothers of teenage daughters.

"Contrary" was a word Frank used often to describe Lucy's stubborn procrastination about helping with chores at times. I remember telling her once, after a particularly hateful, depressing squabble of some kind, "We just can't live like this. We're going to see a psychiatrist or a psychologist or somebody, and find out what's wrong here." At the time I had no idea whether Cookeville even had a psychiatrist. It was simply something I said, but I did have a feeling of foreboding, of things getting out of hand.

Frank left for Atlanta on Thursday, June 15, 1978. I don't recall clearly the jumbled events of that day, but I noticed that Lucy was in her room a lot. We usually ate the evening meal early, between four and five o'clock. I had fixed the food and asked Mark, "Where is Lucy? It's time to eat supper."

"She's been in her room all day listening to the radio," he answered. The song she listened for over and over at that time was Billy Joel's "Only The Good Die Young."

I was concerned about her withdrawal but not frightened. Teenagers are all unfathomable at times. She was usually hungry at mealtime, though, and I went to her room to see why she hadn't come out to eat.

She was sitting in a rocking chair. She was wearing a new red dress, pantyhose, and high heels. I was surprised at this dress-up outfit on an average weekday at home.

"Why are you all dressed up, Lucy? Put on something comfortable and come on out." She just looked at me and continued rocking. "Why are you wearing hose and your new dress?" I asked again. I found her answer incredible.

"Because I'm going to die."

I searched her face in stunned silence, wondering if I had heard her clearly, whether she was just joking, or playing some sort of game. I was tired and hungry and not in the mood for whatever she had in mind. "Now stop talking like that and take off those good clothes. Supper's getting cold," I said.

Her next words were even more jarring. "I told you, I'm going to die. Didn't you hear it on the radio?" She wasn't smiling, and my heart skipped a beat or two. I was still more frustrated than frightened, and I was getting a little irritated at her bewildering behavior.

I thought she might be saying something perverse just to get my attention.

"Lucy, stop talking silly. Hang up your good dress and come on. Let's go eat supper now," I said once more.

She continued rocking, a fixed expression in her eyes, a stubborn, unsmiling look on her face that sent a shock of fear through me. "I told you," she said again, "I'm going to die. It's been on the radio all day."

"Lucy, stop talking like that," I said in a louder, more demanding tone, feeling more anxious at my inability to break through her unnatural spell. "Lucy!" I yelled. "Stop this right now!"

She simply looked at me, and something about her eyes told me not to pursue it further. I knew in that instant that no insistence on my part was going to change anything. I knew beyond a shadow of doubt that something was very wrong, but I had no idea what it was or how to handle it.

The rest of that terrible day when Lucy first became ill is almost lost to me. I have no memory at all of what Frankie and Mark were doing or whether I talked to them. I think it was the following day, Friday, that I called a friend from church and asked her to stop by.

"Something's wrong with Lucy," I told Jenny on the telephone, not elaborating further. I remember waiting and watching for her car and how glad I was when it finally pulled up that afternoon. I walked outside to meet her and said, "Lucy is acting strange. She's watching television in the den now. See if you can talk to her and what you think."

Jenny went into the combination den-kitchen that opened onto a screened porch in back of our house, and I stayed out of the way while they talked. Jenny knew Lucy from their church and Sunday school work together. She is an understanding, accepting person, the kind I desperately needed that day.

Later, Lucy went back to her room, wearing a peculiar smile I had noticed earlier. Jenny and I sat in a utility room near the kitchen and talked. I don't know all the things we spoke of, but before she left, she said, "I think it's serious. I'd talk to Frank, and I think I'd get her to a doctor." She mentioned another friend from church and said, "I know she'll do anything she can to help you get a doctor to see Lucy."

A pall had been thrown over everything in my life. Frank was due back from his Atlanta trip that evening, and I waited tensely, listening for the sound of his car driving in. As soon as I saw the station wagon pulling into our backyard drive, I went out to meet it. "Something's happened to Lucy," I told him through the car window. "Something's wrong with her mind."

Frank, tired from his drive, just looked at me, carried his suitcase inside, and tried to understand what seemed incomprehensible.

Lucy's movements had become stiff, almost robot-like. Her fleeting, odd little smiles at the wrong times had grown into full-blown laughter. She laughed uproariously at practically everything we said. She seemed to be in a totally different world. The symptoms were similar to those of someone on drugs. I never thought of that possibility until we were asked about it at the mental health center later. The tests they did confirmed there was no evidence of drug use. I felt something was slipping irrevocably out of control, and that we were powerless to stop it.

We finally fell into a short sleep that night after giving Lucy some aspirin, hoping it would calm her restless movements. She had tried to stop the hands of, or do something to, our cuckoo clock once early in the evening, and Mark had said, "No, Lucy! Leave it alone—you'll break it!" His voice sounded frightened because her movements were so mechanical, as if she were moving in a dream, propelled by forces we couldn't imagine. I know now how terrible that weekend must have been for Mark and Frankie. I was so overwhelmed by what had happened that I was hardly aware of them at the time.

Something awakened me about two o'clock Saturday morning, and I went to Lucy's room, which was next to ours, to see how she was. The bed was empty. My heart thumped in alarm as I went from room to room and looked outside in the darkened yard. She was nowhere inside or out that I could see. I shook Frank from sleep and told him, "Lucy's not in her room!" We searched the house again and looked outside. "She must be walking down the road," I said. "We've got to find her."

We pulled on clothes and got in the car. We had seen a trail of torn paper in our driveway leading toward the street, and as we backed out in front of the house, Frank said, "Look. Look at the mailbox." Ours, and every other mailbox and newspaper box along the street that led from our house to a main street running east to west ahead, was bent forward.

We followed the trail of bent-over mailboxes along the quiet street, driving slowly, trying to keep panic at bay, not knowing what to expect. Lucy told us later when we asked about it that she had bent over the mailboxes because she wanted to "straighten up the world."

I knew she must be wearing her thin, sleeveless, short nightgown because it wasn't in her empty room. We didn't know which way to turn when we reached the intersection, but we took a chance and turned east toward town. About halfway up a hill we saw her walking on the edge of the road. The sight of her in that little short nightgown on the dark road shoulder is etched in my mind forever. Frank slowed and we pulled up beside her.

"Lucy—Lucy, get in the car, honey," I said, wondering if she would. She stared at us blankly for a moment and then climbed obediently into the backseat and sat near the window. She seemed to be mentally engrossed in unfathomable thoughts. I turned in the seat and asked gently, "What have you been doing?"

"I'm Mary, the mother of Jesus. I'm pregnant. I'm going to give birth to the baby Jesus," she answered and fell back into silence. Frank and I sat mute, numb with shock.

We were filled with thankfulness that we had found her. I kept thinking of the terrible things that might have happened to her that night, being kidnapped, raped, or murdered, perhaps disappearing forever. We were also glad that the police had not spotted her and taken her to the station.

Sometime Sunday morning we took a ride to our farm with my half-brother, Bill, and sister-in-law, Emily, who had stopped for a brief visit sometime over the weekend. I think we all hoped the drive would have a normalizing effect on Lucy. "It will do her good," Emily said as we got into the car. I still thought that Lucy would surely snap back into reality at some point and become herself again.

My journal entry for that Sunday morning reads, "Everything here is changed since Thursday when Lucy began to slip away from us mentally."

Our house during those three days was full of silent weeping. Frank and I cried whenever we heard Lucy laughing in her room. Bill and Emily wept with us. We couldn't seem to talk to each other; we just exchanged glances of mute despair. I noticed that Frankie's eyes were full of tears at one point. I took him aside to talk and discovered his grief was double; he had just broken up with his first girlfriend. I don't remember what was going on with Mark at all.

Lucy laughed continually on our drive to the farm. Once there, Frank started showing Bill and Emily through the almost-finished house, and I stayed with Lucy. I had trouble keeping her from taking off at a brisk walk across the open fields. She seemed to be filled with enormous energy and a need for constant motion. I persuaded her to come back inside the house, found Frank, and whispered desperately, "We've got to get her back to town and to a doctor—now!"

We drove home in a fog of anxiety. Lucy sat in back with Bill and Emily and laughed loudly at our few attempts at conversation. After some anxious telephone calls and the help of a friend from church in getting a doctor on Sunday, we left with Lucy for an emergency appointment at the hospital, relieved that she was willing to go.

After the briefest talk and examination, the doctor made arrangements for her to be admitted to the local mental health center. We drove Lucy out to the unfamiliar facility, a modern, one-story, spreading structure that we'd hardly known was there. It was to become almost a second home to us in the years ahead.

The nurse in charge at Plateau Mental Health Center got Lucy signed in and asked us to stay and give a brief history of what had happened. We told her every detail we could remember from Thursday on.

We were told we could not visit her for three days. Before we left, I asked a nurse at the desk, "Is she still laughing?" She nodded silently.

We drove home, exhausted, filled with bewilderment, shock, and grief but vastly relieved for the moment that she was safe. Sometime during our interview at Plateau a nurse had said, "She's very sick." The words were hard to believe.

Chapter Six

JULY 1978 – JANUARY 1980

"Help Me Fit Into The World"

Whatever else was going through Lucy's mind during those days preceding her break with reality on Thursday, June 15, 1978, religious thoughts played a part. Her psychiatrist at that time assured us that if it had not been religion, it would have been something else, something her mind became obsessed with.

When we looked into her room after taking her to the mental health center that first weekend, Frank and I found a wastebasket full of crumpled papers—pages and pages of prayers. There were lists of almost every friend, relative, and passing acquaintance who had ever been a part of our lives. Apparently Lucy was trying to pray for them all.

One prayer, written on a sheet of notebook paper like the rest, was for herself. It read, "Dear Lord Jesus, please help me fit into the world." Those words are seared into my heart forever. To me, they speak eloquently of Lucy's struggle to find a footing, something to hold back the slide into chronic chaos and confinement that awaited her ahead.

We couldn't visit Lucy for three days. We spent them calling the mental health center, trying to find out exactly what was wrong with her and how she was responding. That information was hard to come by. I wanted to speak to the psychiatrist who was attending her, but we were told, "You can't talk to the psychiatrist." We were assigned to a social worker and told to speak with him about our concerns. Talking to the social worker did not put our anxiety to rest. I called the center frequently, and finally, Lucy's psychiatrist telephoned us.

I remember standing at the kitchen counter, listening with strained intensity to that conversation. I don't know what I expected to hear. I think I believed the doctor would tell me that Lucy had suffered some kind of breakdown but that she would probably be all right in a few days, that he wanted to talk with us about her, that this was not an uncommon thing for those her age.

What he said was, "I think your daughter has had a schizophrenic breakdown." He went on to explain the different types of schizophrenia and the prognosis for improvement for each, but my mind had gone blank. All I heard was the word schizophrenia, a word that jolted my mind with fear as nothing else ever had. Scenes from old magazines with articles about mental illness came to mind, pictures of half-clothed people sitting around like zombies, locked away in dismal-looking halls. I cried for days.

It still seemed incredible that a part of Lucy's mind had gone from us, and we had no idea how to call it back. I was a little relieved to know there was a cause for the problems she had had communicating with people and her sometimes puzzling behavior. I made no note of the diagnosis of schizophrenia in my journal of that period, and it was years before I could say the word openly to people. I don't know when that sinister word became a part of our everyday vocabulary. It had already become a huge part of our lives.

I told the neighbors (the social worker had suggested this) that Lucy had suffered some kind of nervous breakdown and that we weren't sure how long she would be at Plateau Mental Health Center. I was too frightened to say much to anyone, afraid anything I said might cause people to shun Lucy or to make what had happened worse by too much talk.

Lucy was hospitalized about four weeks that first time, and seemed to make a rapid recovery after treatment with antipsychotic drugs. My journal for July 10 reads, "Today Lucy was discharged from Plateau Mental Health and is sleeping on her new Sears mattress that came in today. She is still very tired, but we hope she'll feel like being more active tomorrow. Anyway, am glad she is home. She hated going back yesterday (she had been on a short leave) even though everyone there was very kind and good to her."

She came home with a strange new medicine. I think it was Haldol (haloperidol), one of the older antipsychotic drugs. We had received only sketchy information from Plateau personnel about the real nature of Lucy's illness. She seemed to be her old self. The unreality was gone, and I thought that with good care and support from us, she would be all right. I believed the ugly shadow schizophrenia had cast over us would gradually fade away. The destructive potential of the illness was unthinkable to us at that time.

Lucy's first weeks at home were hard. The medicine made her lethargic and uncomfortable. She had never complained much, but she kept telling me, "Mom, I just don't feel good. I don't want to do anything. Just let me lie here." I couldn't believe it was normal for her to spend most of her time in bed and I made repeated calls to Plateau complaining about her loss of energy and stiff, rigid movements. I was told she was experiencing the normal effects of the medicine, but I finally got an appointment with her psychiatrist.

"She's having a toxic reaction to the medicine," he told us after seeing Lucy one afternoon. He changed her to another antipsychotic drug that she tolerated better, but she stayed in her room a lot and seemed depressed. My journal for July 20 reads, "Lucy had a much better day than yesterday and very happy about that. We did exercises, she helped clean her room, watered some plants, started on a piece of embroidery again, and in general, much more up than down."

One day, not too long after her breakdown, I heard a thumping, banging sound in Lucy's room and hurried, heart pounding, to see what it was about. I opened her bedroom door and asked, "What on earth is going on?" My question caught her with a familiar, tormented expression in her blue eyes as she lay on her rumpled bed. She had been banging a book over and over against the wall. I remember her fierce, frustrated tears, and I can still hear her words, "It keeps running through my head, it keeps running through my head, it keeps running through my *head!*"

I had had phrases and words and sometimes songs drumming

through my brain at times, but eventually they would fade and life went on. "What keeps running through your head?" I asked, trying to understand the cause of her intense distress.

"Honey priss," she answered, two senseless words that kept repeating themselves over and over in her mind. I remember finding her in tears a number of times as she struggled with the maddening recurrence of the words.

I felt helpless and frustrated myself as I tried to understand her problem. But I didn't. I thought, Why can't she get her mind on something else, like cleaning her room, taking a walk, riding her bike, and maybe it won't run through her head. I had no idea then of the mental hell that was beginning to take shape for Lucy.

The summer of 1978 was one of back-breaking work and mental strain for all of us. Lucy helped as we finished work on the farmhouse, sold our house in town, and made the move to the country in September.

School started again and Lucy went back to senior high full of anxiety and fears about her ability to go on. We talked with a school counselor who was very understanding and discovered that she had almost enough credits to graduate already. She finished her high school work that December, graduating with honors, and decided to go to Tennessee Tech for the winter quarter that began in January. She took the American College Test (ACT) in October and scored high in English and math and low in social studies and natural sciences. I was surprised that the test indicated her interest inventory in technical subjects was especially high.

When she was a sophomore in high school, she wrote in front of her yearbook in a large, generous, vertical, rounded hand, "Lucy Holloway, grade 10, age 16 at time of receiving this yearbook." On the page with her picture, she signed her name again with a wide, circular flourish after the "y" in Holloway.

She was very happy with the signatures she collected from classmates at that time: "Lucy, you're really a great girl, and I hope we'll always be friends. I'm looking forward to walking with you in the walk-a-thon. Good luck in the future and God Bless ya!" (Lucy was part of the March of Dimes walkathon in April, 1977). Another classmate wrote, "Lucy, I expect to see you on Broadway! (We'll be a duet of some kind.) You are definitely an angel, and we need more girls like you! My motto 'search for the castles in the clouds (Heaven), stay cool, and strive hard,' God be with ya! Love ya lots!"

Only four classmates wrote somewhat lengthy messages in her senior class yearbook, and she had only a scattering of signatures in her university yearbook in 1981.

Our five years at the farm, "on the mountain," were fleeting and full of activity. They were the last years we were all together as a family. Only Max, our cat, remains of the pets we had there, which included chickens, two donkeys, and two dogs.

Frankie commuted to Tennessee Tech and Mark and Lucy rode to senior high with their father in the fall of 1978. Lucy practiced driving again. I picked her up after school, and she drove our station wagon up the mountain every afternoon. I was still uncomfortable with her driving since she was easily distracted. She drove off the road into a muddy bog near our driveway one afternoon because she said the sun got in her eyes. A neighbor pulled us out, but Lucy wasn't as interested in driving after that, and I was relieved.

A journal note in December reads, "Lucy is working on a long term paper and speech she has to get finished this weekend. She may go to Christmas dance next weekend. Will have to get her a long dress if she does. I can't believe it's her last week at senior high!" I had hoped Lucy would be going to the dance, but it turned out to be another of the disappointments she was almost used to by then. I think some classmates had jokingly suggested she go with a boy they knew, but the invitation didn't come and she didn't go. She passed up going to a play that Mark was in that month too, but we had a nice Christmas together.

Right after Christmas, Frank and I took Lucy and Mark for a week's vacation to Florida. Frankie was working, so he stayed home to look after the house and pets. We stopped at Myrtle Beach and visited relatives in Tallahassee. It was a nice break before a return to school in January.

On January 2, 1979, I wrote, "Frank just left few minutes ago in blowing snow flurries and freezing temperatures. It's Lucy's big day—registration for her first quarter at Tech, and the weather would have to turn fiendish." I don't think Lucy would ever have made the two years she finished at Tennessee Tech without her father's constant support and guidance. Being on campus, he was available when she needed him, and she soon learned her way around the campus that seemed so overwhelming to her at first.

She finished winter and spring quarters that first year with good grades, and she and I took a bus trip to Maryland that June to visit relatives. I am grateful for that trip. I remember we sat up most of the night on the bus. We talked, ate hot dogs for breakfast in the Washington DC station, and had a happy visit with my relatives who had never met Lucy. She was not completely her old self, but her symptoms were mild, her spirits were high, and I was full of hope for her complete recovery.

When we returned, Lucy went back to Tech for the summer quarter. She was pleased with her grades, and we thought she was doing very well. She started her fourth quarter in September, but it did not go smoothly. She suffered almost constant mood swings and anxieties of all kinds. She had started out to major in business administration, but decided to change to dietitian. "I've never been interested in business," she said, and we thought the change would be good as she was interested in food and nutrition.

She had been going to a weekly InterVarsity Bible study group that meant a great deal to her then, and for the next two years, but in mid-December she told me one evening, "I don't want to go to Bible study tonight. I'm afraid I'll start laughing." This inappropriate laughter was one of the symptoms that plagued Lucy whenever she began to lose control. She was also extremely restless and unable to relax. On December 14, I wrote, "Cold and fair. Lucy and I cleaned house and washed clothes yesterday while it rained off and on. She is not feeling too good (laughing) and didn't go to Bible study last night. Hope she can see Dr. Johnson Monday if not better."

She suffered a second breakdown on December 16, 1979, at age eighteen, in the middle of her second year at Tech. The details are hazy, but I remember Lucy had been getting more and more out of touch with reality for several days. That evening, things came completely unraveled. She and I were alone in the house. Frankie must have been working, and Frank had taken Mark into town to practice for a Christmas play at our church. Lucy had been talking and moving constantly, saying things that made no sense to me and growing very irritated with whatever comment I made in response.

"What are you looking at me like that for?" she asked, noting my increasing nervousness. I was afraid to say much of anything for fear it would make things worse. I thought Frank and Mark would never get home, and as soon as they walked in the door, I told Frank, "We've got to get Lucy to the hospital."

I am sure that Lucy was taking her medicine during this period. She complained about the drugs frequently, but she had been on antipsychotic medications since her breakdown in June of 1978, and had never refused to take them. "It's not fair," she told me once. "I have to take all this medicine just to be normal." I agreed and longed for a time when she could be free of the drugs.

She readily agreed to Frank's suggestion that we go for a drive to look at the Christmas lights in town that night. I recall driving down the mountain, chattering about the lights of Cookeville in the distance, while my mind whirled with questions. Would Lucy mind our stopping at the hospital? Would she go inside to see a doctor?

It all went smoothly after I went into the hospital emergency room and told a nurse, "Our daughter is outside. She's in a psychotic state and needs to see a doctor now." The nurse told me to bring her in, and Lucy was in fine spirits when she walked into the hospital. While we waited a few minutes for the doctor, I noticed her staring at a young man with a dark, shaggy beard and brown, flowing hair who was also waiting. When the nurse summoned us, Lucy paused before this man, gave him a beatific smile, and asked, "Are you Jesus?"

"Come on, Luce," I mumbled, hurrying her past, trying not to imagine what the startled fellow thought of her unusual question.

She was admitted to Plateau Mental Health Center again that evening and spent Christmas there. She came home on leave on Friday, January 11, 1980, and was to be discharged the following Friday, January 18. The day before she was to come home, our lives were plunged into trauma once more when I answered a phone call on Thursday afternoon, January 17.

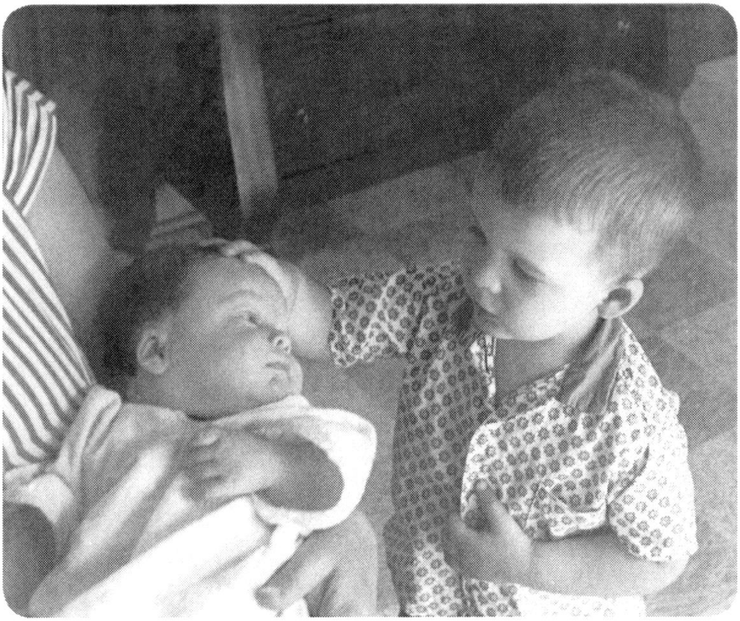

Lucy and Frank, 1961

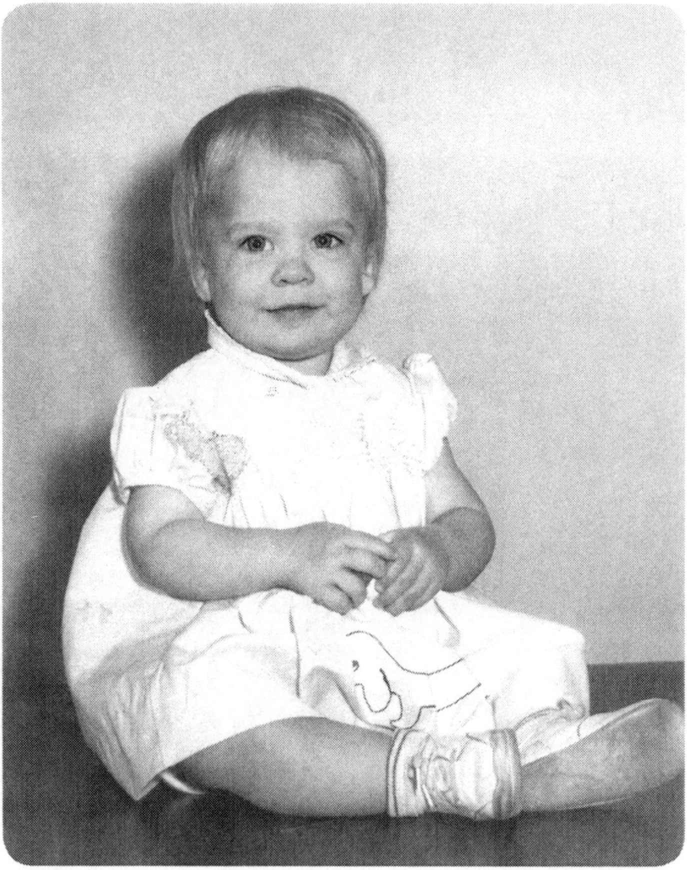

Lucy, Age 1

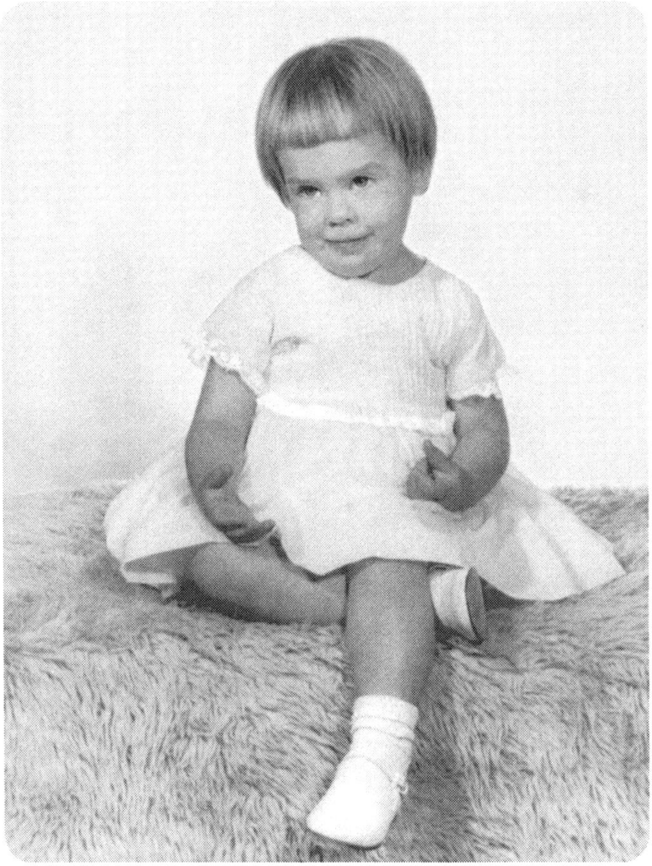

Lucy, Age 2, Tallahassee, Florida

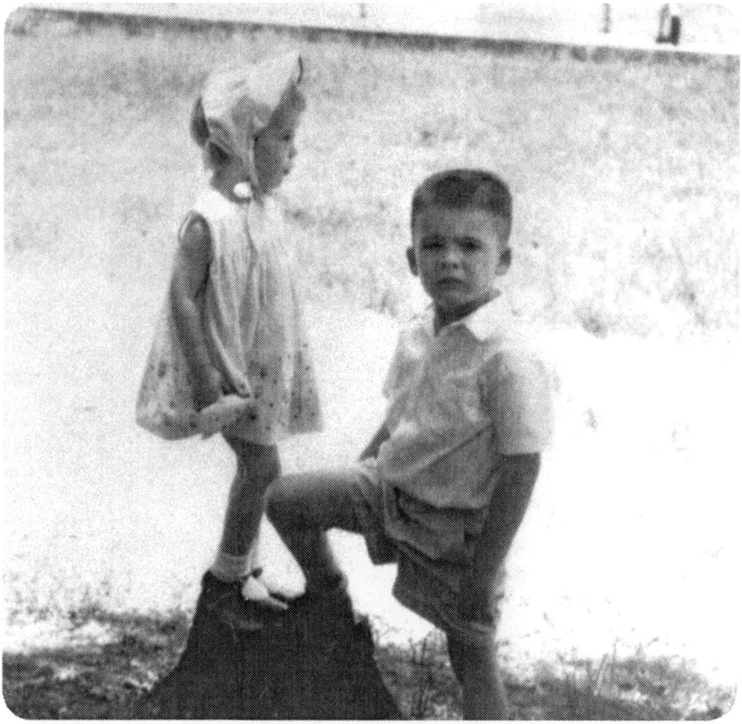

Lucy and Frank, 1960s

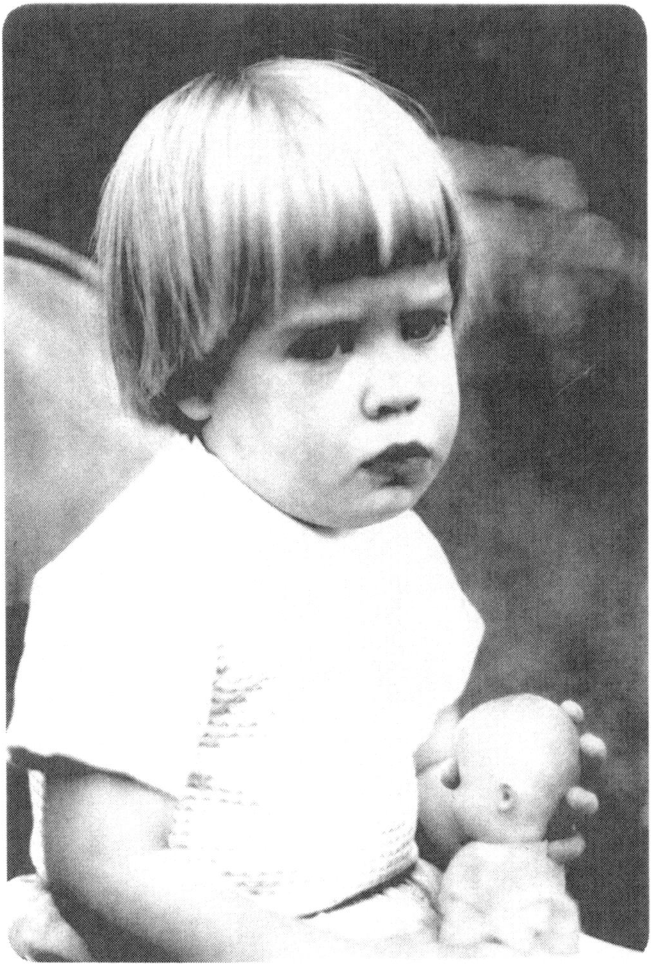

Lucy, Tallahassee, Spring 1963

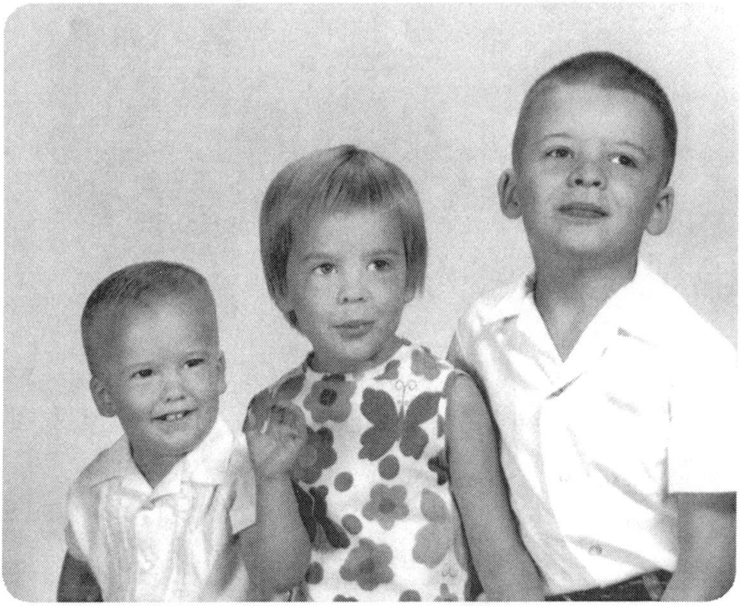

Mark, Lucy, and Frankie – Tallahassee, 1965

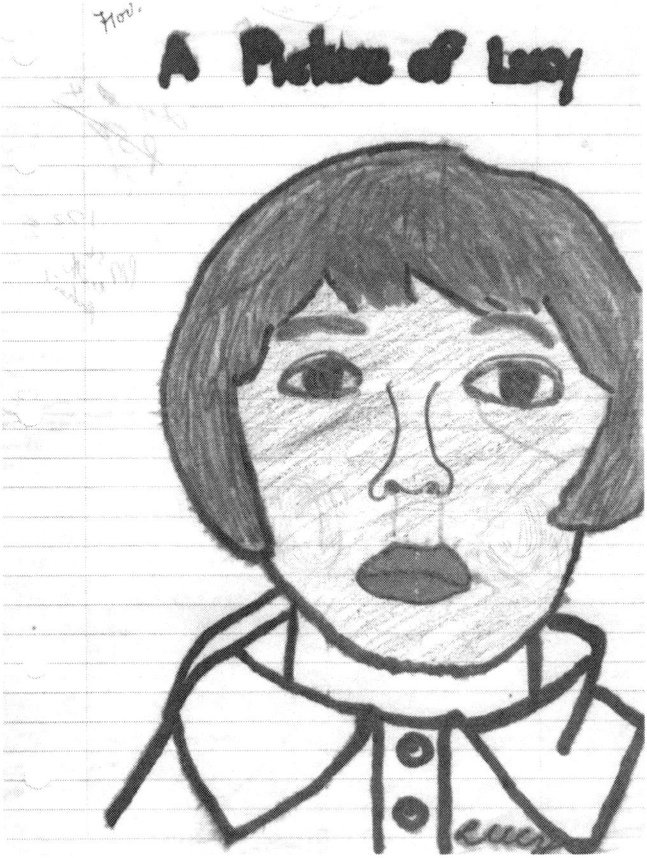

Lucy self-portrait, 1970

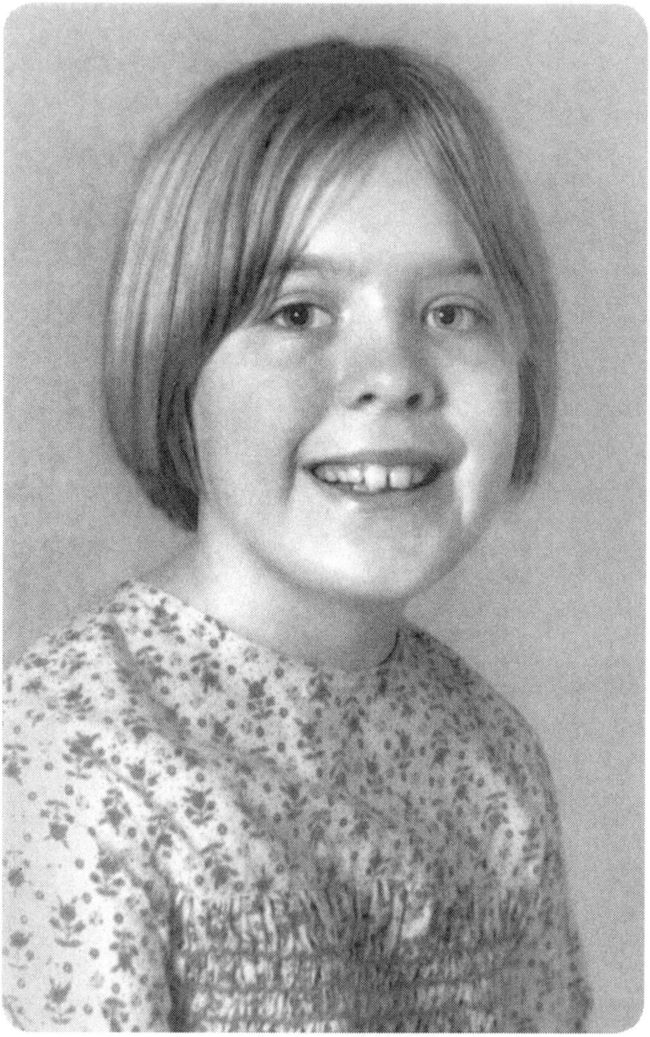

Lucy school portrait, 1972

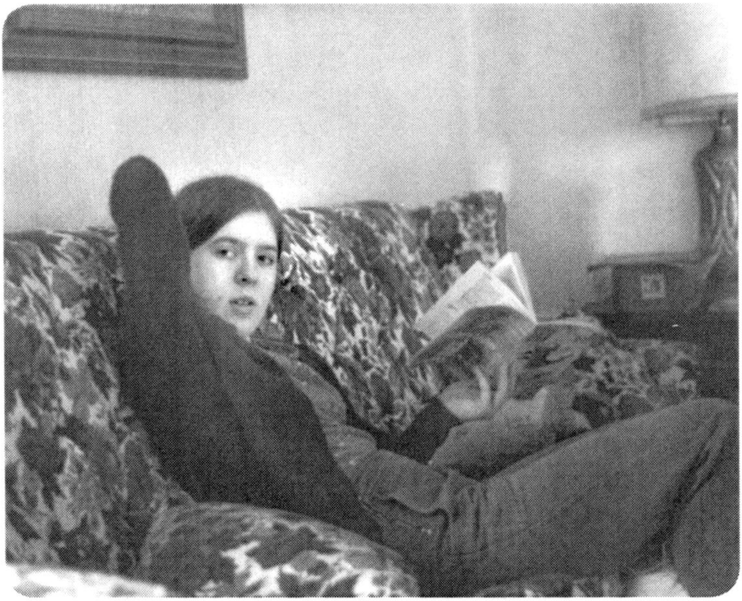

Lucy, 1970s, Cookeville, Tennessee

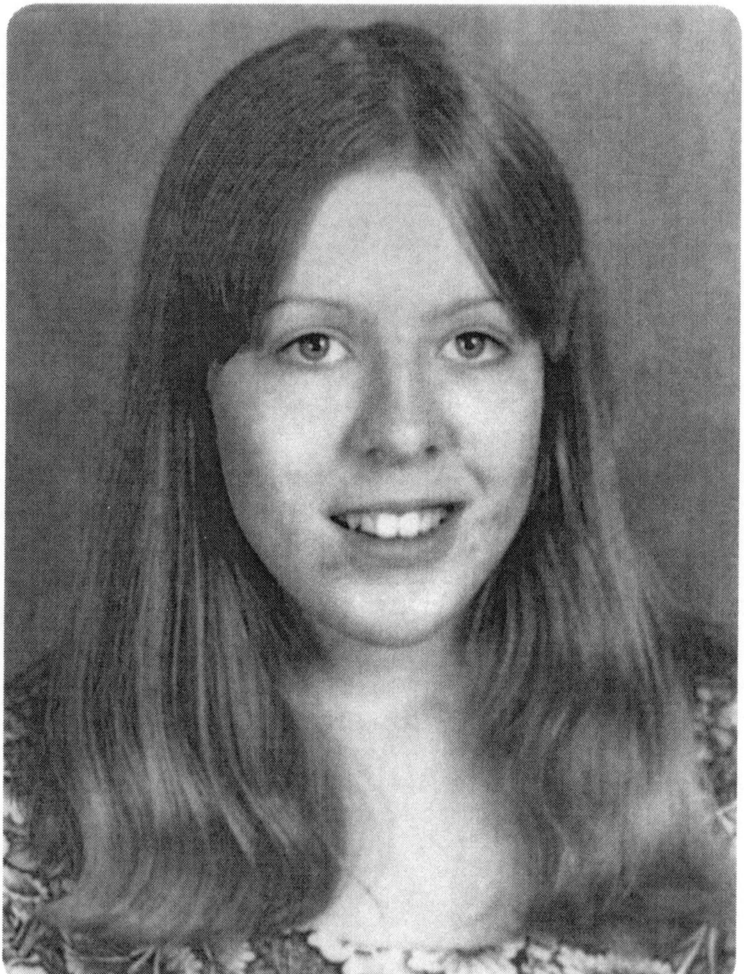

Lucy school portrait, 1975

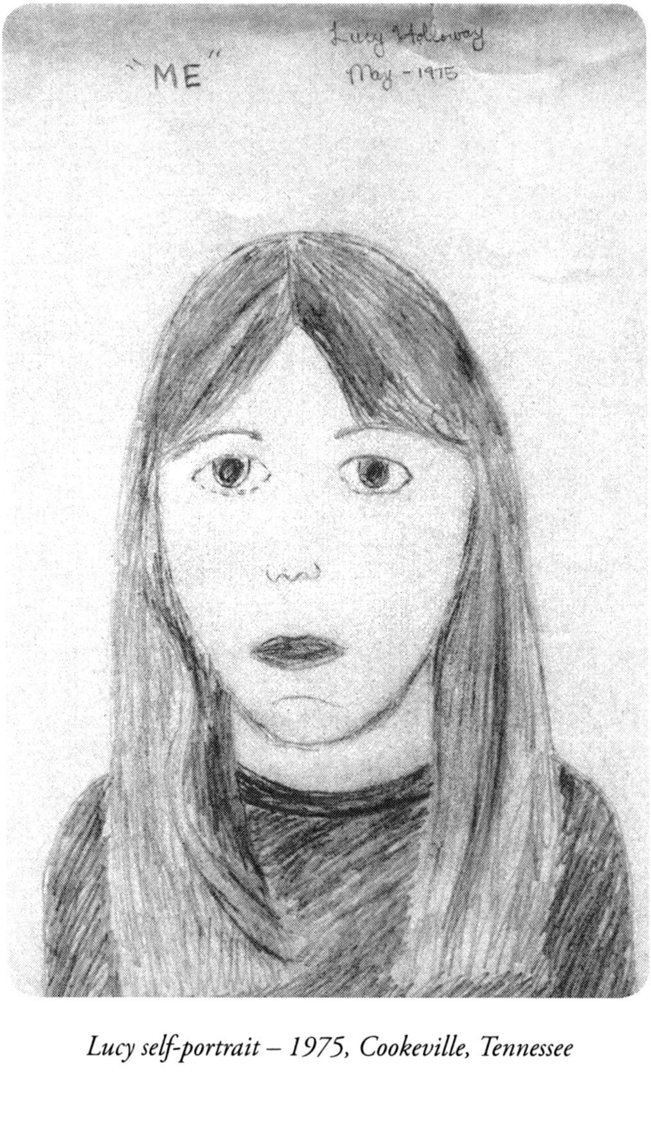

Lucy self-portrait – 1975, Cookeville, Tennessee

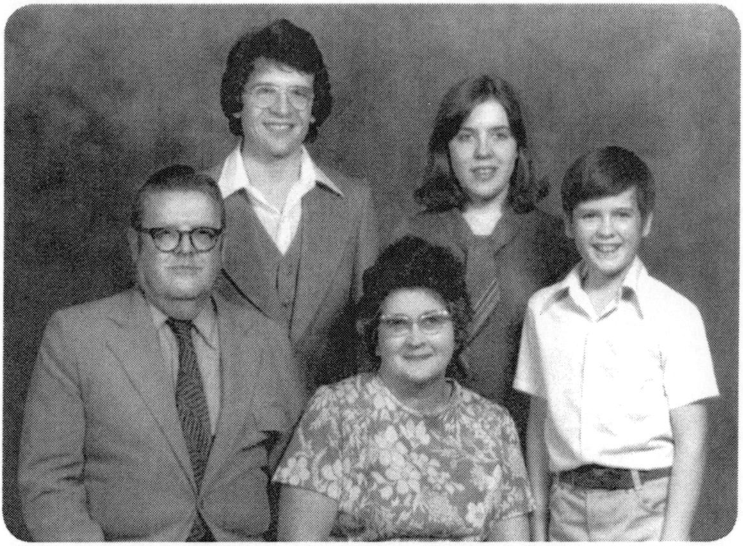

Family portrait, 1977

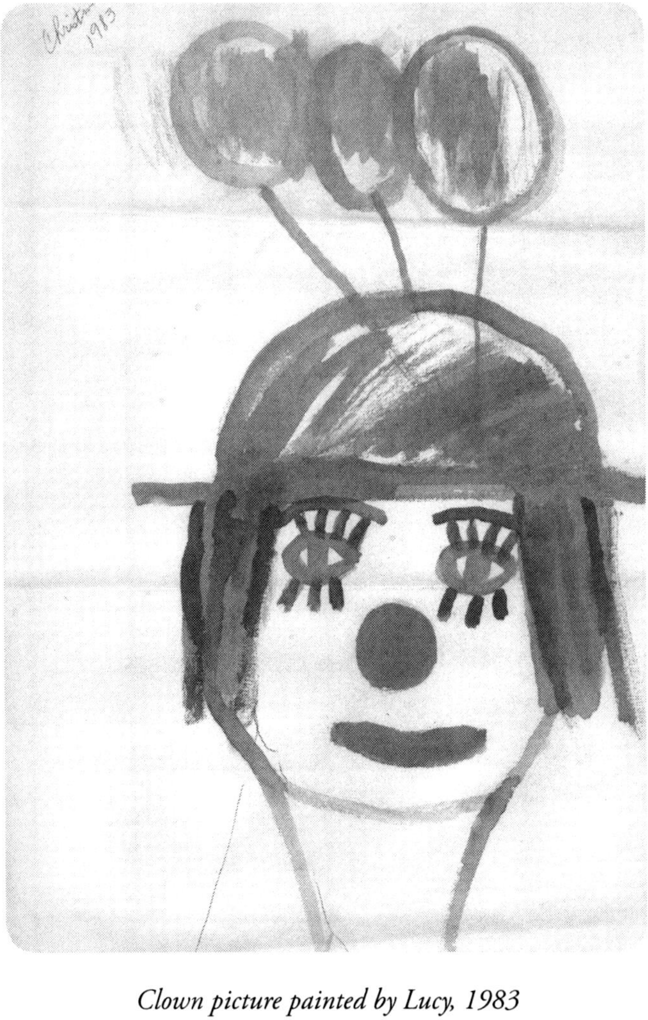

Clown picture painted by Lucy, 1983

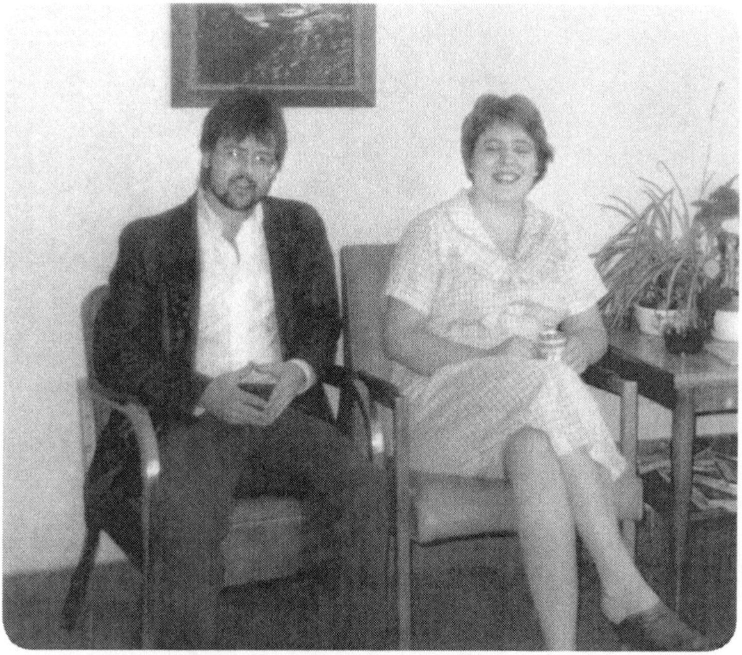

Mark and Lucy at Moccasin Bend, 1984

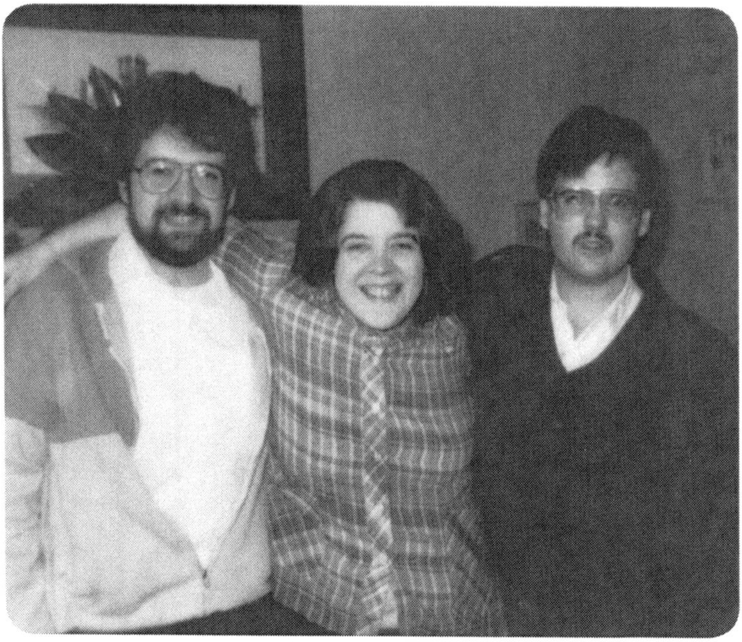

Frankie, Lucy, and Mark, 1985

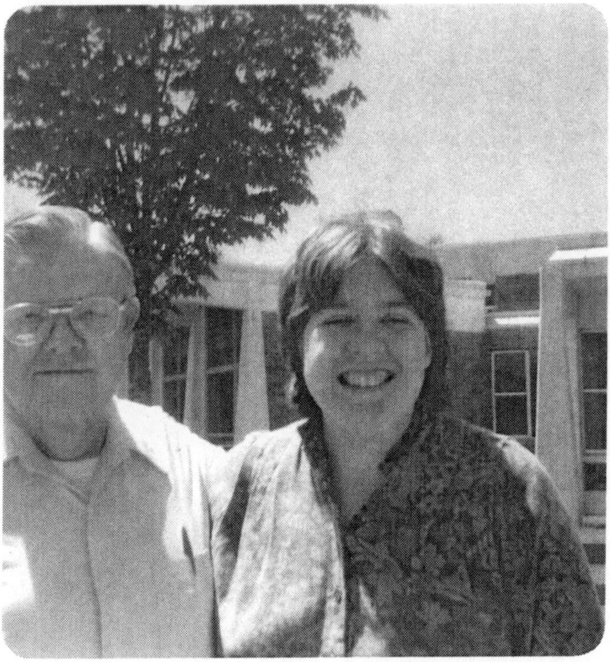

Dad and Lucy at Moccasin Bend, 1985

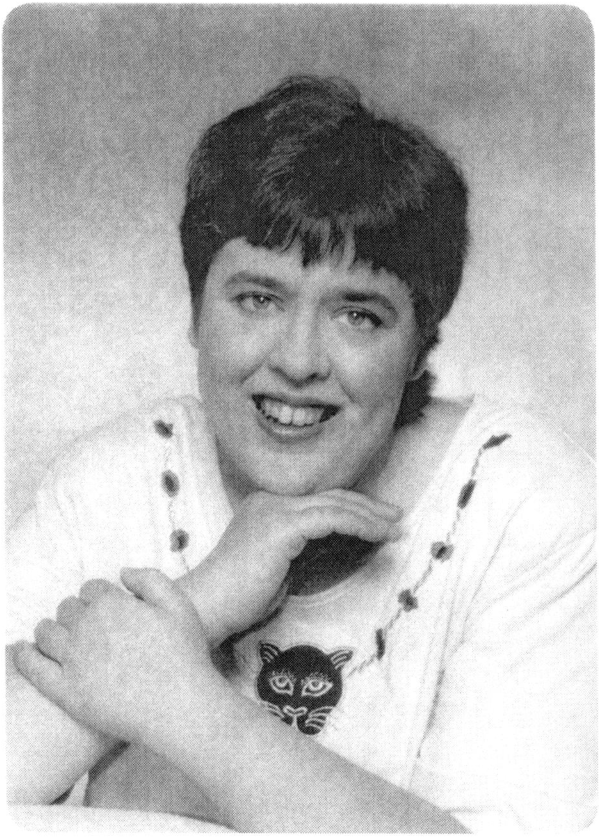

Lucy, 1998

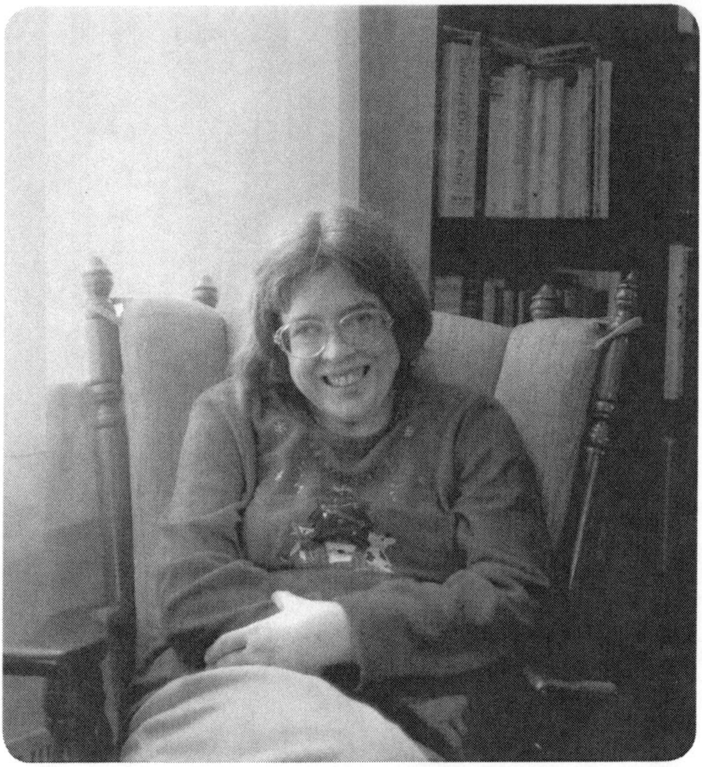

Lucy, Christmas 2004

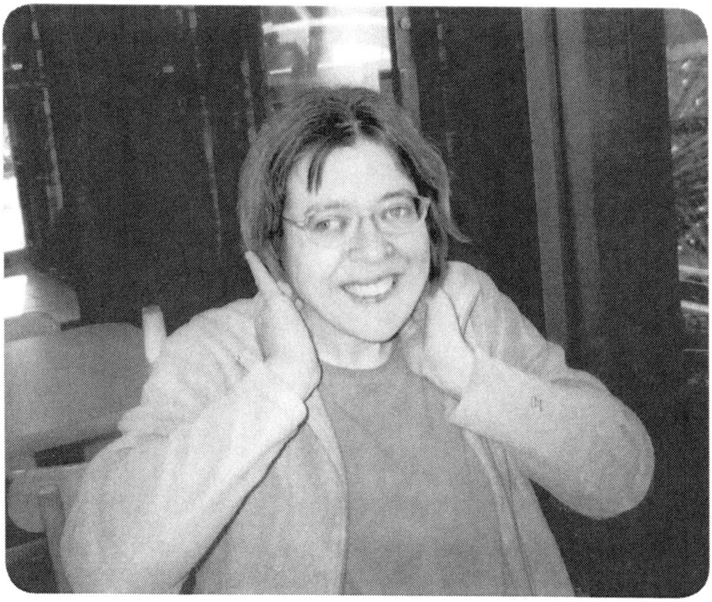

Lucy, 2008

Chapter Seven
JANUARY 1980 – OCTOBER 1982

"She Was Doing So Well"

I wondered which one of the children was calling when the phone rang that drizzly, gray afternoon shortly after the school day had ended. I remember feeling only slightly uneasy when a strange male voice informed me, "Your son's been involved in an accident, and you and your husband had better get on down to the hospital."

"Is he hurt bad?" I asked, assuming he was talking about Frankie because Mark was not driving at that time.

"I don't think it's too bad," he answered, "but you and your husband had better come on down here. You need to be at the hospital," he said again with a strange insistence.

I hurriedly telephoned Frank at the university, and he said he would go to the hospital. I still thought the accident was just a fender-bender involving our oldest son. I imagined they were patching him up and just needed one of us to take him home from the hospital. I wasn't sure that I would even be needed as I waited for Frank to call me from the emergency room. But my life had gone on hold, suspended until I knew things were all right again.

It seemed like hours before Frank called. "You need to come on to the emergency room," he said in a calm but strained voice as soon as I lifted the receiver. "Mark and two friends have been in a serious accident. The other families and some friends are already here."

"How bad is he hurt?" I asked, as a feeling of dread began to envelop me.

"I'm still waiting for a report, and I'm going to call our doctor," he answered, adding, "I can't get any information here."

The full impact of the accident didn't sink in until hours later in the emergency room of Vanderbilt Hospital in Nashville. Soon after I arrived at Cookeville General Hospital, I learned that Mark's two classmates were being transferred to Vanderbilt, both with critical injuries. A short while later, after our family doctor had examined Mark, he came out to us and said, "I think Mark needs to go to Vanderbilt, too." We learned later that our doctor had recognized Mark was in a coma and insisted that he be sent to Vanderbilt, an act we felt might have saved his life. Frank and I hastily conferred and decided I would go in the ambulance with Mark and he would stay home to see about Lucy, who was due home from Plateau the next day.

All three children had suffered critical head injuries, and one of them, Mark's best friend at the time, who had just turned sixteen, died a week later. Mark and his other classmate remained at Vanderbilt for weeks, slowly recovering from extensive injuries.

Mark remained in a coma for about seven days, staring at us blankly when we went in to visit and talk to him at the scheduled hours. We wondered if he would ever regain total awareness.

Gradually, he began talking and eating again, ultimately making an almost miraculous recovery physically.

We were constantly supported and comforted by the prayers of distant relatives and those of friends in Cookeville and at the hospital during that time. Without them, we could not have borne the grief and pain of those days, which we shared with the other two families involved.

Throughout the following year, Mark got good physical reports from his neurosurgeon in Nashville when we went for scheduled checkups. He began suffering from anxiety and depression during his junior year in high school in the fall and winter of 1980-1981. These symptoms blossomed into a full-fledged psychosis in 1983 when he was diagnosed as having a bipolar or manic-depressive illness, which continues to the present.

There is no way of knowing, but we think Mark may never have developed a serious psychosis if it had not been for the accident. His story would require another book, and I mention his illness here because he and Lucy suffered a number of overlapping periods of illness and hospitalization from 1980 to 1986.

Lucy came home from Plateau as scheduled after Mark's accident and did very well considering the situation. Friends from her Bible study group and from our church brought food and stayed with her when needed to help Frank. I stayed at the hospital most of the time except weekends when Frank came over. Frankie and Lucy both visited, but when Lucy saw Mark, she asked, "Why doesn't he wake up?" We found it hard to explain and realized Lucy's comprehensive abilities had changed.

She was doing well at the time, however, and started back to Tennessee Tech for the spring quarter in March 1980. She was nineteen that month, and we celebrated with burgers and fries at McDonald's.

Some of our best days during the years from 1979 to 1982 were when Lucy and I attended an InterVarsity Bible study group together. I went, a little reluctantly at first, at Lucy's invitation. I've always been grateful for that period. I never imagined that those often stressful days might be the best and most functional ones Lucy would have.

Some of the friends Lucy knew at Bible study and some from our church, as well as my daughter-in-law, will always have a special place in my heart because of the patience and love they showed to Lucy during the years of her growing confusion. She talked to some of them by the hour on the telephone and called frequently, especially during the times she was feeling the worst. The telephone was her lifeline.

Lucy called her friends, but the telephone rarely rang for her. She often ran to answer it; when it was for another family member and would say, "It's not fair! Nobody ever calls me!" I felt her disappointment and isolation keenly and wished for one person who would just call her regularly and say "hello." I also felt embarrassed at times by the loud, lengthy conversations she had when she called others. She seemed to be unaware of any need to moderate the flow of words. I felt the desperation in her sometimes shrill exchanges and worried that it might turn people away from her.

In June of 1980, we took Lucy to Nashville for an evaluation by a private psychiatrist. He only confirmed her local doctor's diagnosis of schizophrenia, and we learned little from the visit. Again, in June of 1981, in another effort to find help for Lucy's continuing anxieties and mood swings, we made an appointment with another psychiatrist in Nashville. We wanted most of all to have an in-depth conference and evaluation of Lucy's condition and the prognosis for improvement. We hoped to learn there was some better medicine or treatment available.

We left Lucy at St. Thomas Hospital in Nashville on June 9, 1981, for a week of observation and evaluation by this psychiatrist. This was during one of Lucy's best periods. She was in good spirits, seemed happy with the hospital, and we were pleased with the caliber of care and attention she received there.

Once again we failed to get much new information and surely not any in-depth conference from the doctor who monitored her stay at St. Thomas. I recall a brief, fifteen-minute talk and got the impression from his remarks that he thought we should have sought help for Lucy much earlier in her life. His comment during the conference, with Lucy present, that she was "socially retarded," or words to that effect, stayed in her mind long after everything positive had faded.

In contrast, the social worker who worked with Lucy at St. Thomas was very encouraging. She talked with Frank and me as if she valued our opinion, which meant a lot, and left us feeling hopeful that things could change for the better.

"Lucy has a lot of strengths," she said, "but she needs help. She has been very responsive in our group here, and we think it would help a lot if she could continue with this. She needs contact with people her own age and help in acquiring better social skills."

I agreed completely with her comments and felt a return of hope that positive changes were within reach. The social worker at St. Thomas talked with the Plateau Mental Health Center staff about arranging for group therapy for Lucy, but when we returned to Cookeville, we found little enthusiasm for the idea at Plateau. Lucy's psychiatrist agreed to have her attend group therapy, but he didn't seem to feel it would do her any good. Lucy attended for a while, but there was nobody in her group that she could identify with; most were older and uncommunicative, and her interest gradually faded.

The summer of 1981 seems peaceful as I look back. It was a blackberry summer on the mountain. We picked tons of berries, froze some and sold some, and put up tomato juice and corn from a bountiful crop in Frank's garden. Lucy helped with garden and housework and seemed to be doing very well overall. A journal note in July reads, "Lucy in very good spirits. Helped indoors, cleaned bathrooms, ironed, and made a delicious batch of oatmeal cookies."

Around the first of August, Lucy began having problems again with mood swings and inappropriate laughter. She suffered a third, totally unexpected, breakdown on August 15. We took her back to Plateau Mental Health Center, and on the way home, Frank and I kept saying to each other, "She was doing so well; she seemed to be doing so well." We were appalled that it had happened again. We went upstairs to her sunny bedroom later, searching for some reason for the relentless return of psychosis.

Her wastebasket overflowed with torn bits of paper that looked like letters she had been writing. I'll never forget my husband's tears and his broken-hearted determination to "find out what's going on in her mind." He started fishing the pieces of paper from the wastebasket, laying them on the bed in an effort to put them together.

"You'll never be able to get them together," I told him. "It's hopeless to try."

But he persisted, placing the pieces like puzzle parts first on Lucy's bed, and later on a table downstairs until he had put together five of the letters. That he was able to do it still seems like a miracle to me, but after he did, none of the sheets made any sense to us. It was like trying to piece together the shattered fragments of her personality. The riddle of schizophrenia remained a dark, impenetrable void.

Lucy improved rapidly after this breakdown and was discharged from Plateau on September 4. On Labor Day, Frank and I decided to go on a picnic to Burgess Falls, a nearby state park, with all of the children. We picked up fried chicken and drinks, and Frank, Frankie, Lucy, and Mark and I were together for the first time in a long while. It was the last picnic Lucy would have with all of us. We walked the trails and took pictures after our lunch. It was a brief, happy time that was not to last.

The fall and winter of 1981 were strained for all of us. Frankie was struggling to hold down a part-time job and keep up his grades at the university, and Mark began suffering suicidal depressions during his senior year at high school. Lucy's anxieties and mood swings seemed to be unending.

I think some of the most tormenting times for Lucy in those early years of her sickness may have been at the farm when she felt the tug of uncontrollable hostility toward me and, to a lesser degree, toward her brothers and father. I remember finding her sobbing in her room, perhaps terrified by the "bad thoughts" that plagued her in a special, hellish way because of her already loosened and scattering control. I remember her telling me with tears of terrible frustration in her eyes, "I think awful things about you—I don't have a conscience—I'm not like other people."

I saw the anguish in her eyes, felt the fear in her cold, sweating palms, and remember her frightened inability to express her inexpressible emotions. A line from Edna St. Vincent Millay's poem "Prayer to Persephone" best describes how Lucy seemed to me in those days.

"…She that had no need of me,
Is a little lonely child
Lost in Hell…"[5]

I wanted so much to comfort and help her then. I don't know how much I did.

When the new year began, Lucy was doing well again. She finished piecing a quilt she had been working on in January and seemed to be getting on well with her classwork at the university. She had grown very distant and uncommunicative toward me that winter. A journal note from the latter part of February reads, "Lucy a little more communicative and am glad. I miss her when she doesn't talk to us."

She had been riding back and forth to classes at Tennessee Tech University with Frankie, and he came into the kitchen one afternoon after they got home to tell me in troubled tones, "Mama, you ought to hear the crazy things Lucy has been saying about you. She told me you tortured her by sticking pins in her when she was a baby, that you'd always hated her. I told her it wasn't true, but it didn't get through at all."

I was stunned and hurt. "Stuck *pins* in her?" The words were incredible. I stared at Frankie in disbelief.

"That's what she's been saying. She insists it's true." He looked at me helplessly, his expression mirroring concern and at the same time, conveying his own message of frustration: I've got to study; I can't handle this kind of stuff.

I had trouble thinking of Lucy's hostility toward me during this period as being connected with her illness. Her accusation was incomprehensible, and I took it personally. I called her downstairs to the kitchen and confronted her angrily. "What have you been telling Frankie about me sticking pins in you when you were a baby?"

She looked at me with the sullen, hooded hostility I'd come to expect at that time and answered unhesitatingly, "It's true. You've always hated me and picked on me because you had a hard time when I was born."

"That's just a plain lie, and don't you ever say such things again," I told her, seething at her insistence on the story.

She turned and went back up the stairs without further comment, but her hostility and remoteness from me continued and ended in one of her worst breakdowns on February 25, 1982. I will always wonder if something happened to her at the university that day that precipitated the break.

She had come home from school in the afternoon with my husband, and I heard her crying loudly as they came through the door. "What's the matter with Lucy?" I asked Frank, watching worriedly as she mounted the stairs with a stack of books.

"I don't know," he said, with a bewildered look. "She just started crying as soon as she got in the car. I couldn't get a word out of her."

I hurried up the stairs to her room and put my arms around her. "What's the matter, Luce? Don't cry. Tell me what's wrong." She clung to me and continued sobbing. "Please, Lucy, tell me what happened. Did somebody hurt you at school? Tell me what happened."

She finally grew quieter, but her eyes were strange and haunted looking. She looked deeply into my eyes once and said, "I can't tell you." Then she added, "Somebody said I was a bitch," and began weeping bitterly again.

From that moment, Lucy went quickly downhill into what seemed to be an almost catatonic psychotic state by the following day when we finally got her hospitalized at the local mental health center. She seemed more frightened and remote than I could ever remember seeing her before. I held her hands and found them cold and clammy with perspiration.

When this process began—the slide into psychosis— there was no more peace or rest for any of us until Lucy was hospitalized. Sometimes it was hours, sometimes days. We knew it was coming, but there was only the helplessness of being sucked into a gathering vortex, trying desperately to hold back the forces that were taking over her mind. There were increasingly desperate calls to the mental health center and calls to the doctor, if we could find one.

I slipped into a room when Lucy wasn't around and called the mental health center. "Lucy isn't doing well at all…I *did* increase the medicine. It doesn't seem to be doing any good…When will the doctor be in?" The crises always seemed to come on weekends or other days when psychiatrists were not at the center. Our frantic questions ("When can she get an appointment? What are we supposed to do?") seemed to fall on deaf ears.

I remember sitting up with Lucy through the night, holding on to her, patting her back, trying to find some way to comfort her, to help her sleep. She was constantly moving or talking, saying things that made no sense.

Frank had gone upstairs to Lucy's room to try to sleep, and I got Lucy to lie down in our room. We were both afraid she might walk out of the house into the night if one of us didn't watch. I lay beside her and prayed over and over, "Lord, please quiet her mind, help her to sleep, comfort her, let this pass…" The prayers seemed empty. I had no feeling that anything made any difference.

It had begun, and we were caught up in an unbearable tension that drew us tighter and tighter as we watched the worsening symptoms: the quickening, agitated, restless movements; the inappropriate laughter getting out of control; and the ever increasing remoteness. We watched helplessly as her mind went spinning out of control almost beyond recall.

When morning finally came, the distant look in Lucy's eyes was frightening. She had periods of being almost completely unreachable. The fear in her eyes was palpable at times. "I'm the devil himself, don't you understand?" she said once. "I'm going to be crucified."

"No, Lucy, no. That's not true," I said, holding her cold, damp hands, trying physically to stop the awful thing that was happening.

We made more urgent calls to Plateau trying to get an appointment, but nobody seemed to realize the critical nature of the situation. Finally a counselor from the center that we knew helped us to break through the seemingly impervious rules to get emergency treatment that day.

Lucy went willingly with us to keep the appointment that afternoon. The doctor who saw her asked in my presence, "How do you feel, Lucy?"

"I feel terrible," she answered.

A short time later we heard the beautiful words, "Lucy, you can go on back. You need to sign some papers." And then, "She's signed in. Bring some clothes out tomorrow. You all get some rest."

Frank and I went home, relieved, but unbearably sad. Now we could sleep, watch television, read, garden, or work for a while in peace, knowing she was safe. At the same time, I felt terrible guilt at my relief when I knew what mental suffering she was going through.

Lucy stayed at Plateau longer than she ever had. As the weeks turned into months, it was hard for us to see much improvement. She spent her twenty-first birthday at Plateau. Frank, Mark, and I took a little cake and went out to see her that evening, but I can't remember how things went for the visit.

Spring was in full bloom when she came home for good on May 14. On Thursday, May 13, I wrote, "Lucy will be home tomorrow from the center for good! I hope she will never have to go back. She'll be going to a day care program three days a week, Monday, Tuesday, and Thursdays, and hope that will be helpful for her. She has been at the center two and a half months, longer than she's ever stayed before. Am hoping she will get interested in some of the animals or something here and not be miserable."

May 1982 was dry and beautiful, as is usual for May in Tennessee. Our strawberries were getting ripe, the Knoxville World's Fair had begun, John Hinckley Jr.'s trial for the attempted assassination of President Reagan was a big news story, and I had recently installed a setting hen on eighteen brown eggs in our new henhouse.

Frankie went to a banquet at the Sheraton Hotel in Nashville for three-star letter writers to the *Tennessean* newspaper, and Mark and some of his friends were in a speech department presentation, *After the Apple*, that played May 7, 8, and 9 at the local drama center. Frank was engrossed in his vegetable garden.

Thursday, May 20 began normally enough. Our small kitchen was bright with spring sunshine and the morning smells of coffee and cooking sausage. Frank was still dressing, our oldest son had left earlier for the university, and Mark was getting ready for senior high school.

I had called up the stairs for Lucy to get up several times that morning. Her scheduled attendance at the day care program at Plateau (a structured period of therapies and crafts from 9 a.m. until 4 p.m. for outpatients) would prove crucial in the day's unfolding events. Getting Lucy up and dressed for day care had been a tug-of-war struggle since the first morning she started.

"I don't need to go to that stupid day care. Please, just leave me alone. I don't get anything out of it. I don't need to go!" she would plead. We thought the structured time might be helpful to her and insisted that she try it for a while.

Frank would drop Mark off at the high school on his way to work while I took Lucy to Plateau, trying to leave by 8:30 for the twenty-mile round-trip. I listened again for sounds of stirring in Lucy's room, which was directly over our kitchen. Hearing nothing, I shouted up the stairs, "Lucy, get up! You have to get ready. You know we have to leave here before nine."

There was no answer, but suddenly she hurried down the stairs and into the kitchen, mumbling something I couldn't understand. She went into the dining room, and I went back to the kitchen, trying to remember what chores I had to do that day, and what Mark's and my husband's schedules were. I was getting eggs and sausage cooked and expected Lucy to come in and say she didn't want that for breakfast. She usually chose something other than what I had fixed, but she still hadn't appeared.

I thought she was in the dining room, but a fleeting uneasiness came over me about her hurrying figure and the silence in the adjoining room. I looked through the doorway, but she wasn't there. She wasn't in the living room or in the downstairs bathroom, so I decided she had gone upstairs and gotten back in bed, something she was prone to do.

But she hadn't complained about going that morning; there had been no gripes about breakfast or not having anything to wear. Something didn't seem right. I've come to trust this feeling implicitly in the past several years.

I called up the stairs again, "Lucy, are you up? Don't you want some breakfast?" No answer. I called again, "Lucy!" Feeling irritated, I climbed the stairs to make sure she had gone back up and was dressing. I opened her door and stepped inside. She was in bed, huddled under the covers.

"I'm not going to day care," she said as soon as she saw me.

"Oh, yes you are. Now, you just get up right now. We're leaving here in a few minutes. Now get up, Lucy!"

"I don't feel good today. Please! Just go out and leave me alone. I'm not going to day care." Her familiar, whining tone exasperated me.

"Lucy, you agreed to do this. Now, get up and get dressed," I yelled.

"What's going on up there?" I went out her door and saw Frank at the foot of the stairs, looking up with a frown that said, "What now?"

"She won't get up. Says she's not going to day care."

Frank came upstairs and into Lucy's room and Mark stepped across the hall from his room and joined us. We all converged on Lucy. My husband said, "Lucy, you promised you'd go to day care. Come on and get up."

Mark added, "Lucy, you need to go. It's your responsibility. Come on and get up."

I yanked at her covers. She just lay curled in the bed and looked at us.

"I don't feel good. Just leave me alone."

"Why don't you feel good?" I asked quickly, tingling with vague disquietude again.

"I just don't feel good," she answered, not looking at us.

"*Why* don't you feel good?" I pressed, a gnawing fear taking stronger shape.

"I don't feel good because—I took some pills," she mumbled, and suddenly we were all galvanized, speaking as one, our voices shrill with dread.

"Took some pills? What kind of pills?"

"Lucy! What kind of *pills*?"

"I took those," she said, gesturing toward her trash basket. Mark grabbed a bottle from it and gasped when he saw the label.

"My God, Lucy! This is my medicine. My doctor said it could kill you!"

We kept all pill bottles hidden, but this one had somehow escaped attention. It was Triavil, a potent anti-depressant drug that one doctor had prescribed for Mark, but he had taken it only a few times. I had seen the bottle on the bookcase in the dining room earlier that week and had meant to put it away. Frank had mentioned it, too, and I thought he had put it up with the rest.

We were all talking at once. "Call Dr. Wilson. Call Plateau. Get the emergency room—Oh, my God!"

Lucy lay watching us with dull eyes. "How many did you take, Lucy?" I asked. "How many did you take?"

"I don't know. Just leave me alone."

I got Plateau on the telephone, told them it was an emergency, and was put through to Dr. Wilson, who had prescribed the drug for Mark. He heard me out and said tersely, "Get her to the emergency room right now."

Frank and I helped Lucy up, urging, "Come on, Lucy. Put this on. We've got to get to the hospital. Come on." We helped her into clothes and led her gently down the stairs and into the car. Mark got in the backseat of the station wagon beside her and Frank said, "Don't let her go to sleep, Mark. Keep her awake. Talk to her."

We sped down the mountain road, and I twisted my head to watch her, listening as Mark repeated over and over, "Don't go to sleep, Lucy. Lucy, talk to me! Don't go to sleep, Lucy! Answer me! Don't go to sleep!"

We were hurrying, hurrying, not believing it was happening, but feeling the urgency build with every passing second. Seven miles to town, ten minutes, three minutes more to thread through the short streets to the emergency room of Cookeville General.

By the time we reached the entrance, Mark looked panicky. Lucy's body was getting limp and her speech slurred frighteningly in our ears. "Come on, Lucy, come on. Don't go to sleep." We continued talking as we helped her from the car. Then running figures were taking her through the double doors of the emergency room. I can't remember, but I guess one of us had called the hospital before we left the farm.

Frank and I stood at the desk, filling out papers, answering questions, showing the nurse the awful, empty bottle. We still didn't believe it could be too bad. They'd pump her stomach or something and it would be okay. We sat on the plastic covered chairs and waited. We'd called our doctor and had been told that he was there.

After what seemed eternity, a nurse was saying, "We're not getting any response. Your doctor is having her taken upstairs to intensive care." The words rattled through my head, "Not getting any response, not getting any response…"

"I'd better call somebody," I told Frank, thinking of friends who knew Lucy, of some who would come to wait with us, some who would come to pray with us…

The next twenty-four hours run together in a jumbled collage of images. Friends joined us in the intensive care waiting room during the morning. Frankie, who had been at school, somehow got a message at the home of our future daughter-in-law, and they came to the hospital. I hardly remember seeing them. Somebody took Mark home at some point, and the hours dragged on.

We went into the ICU room at intervals to see Lucy and talked to her as much as we could. She lay, hooked to a respirator, still and unresponsive. For me, it was reliving the old nightmare from 1980 when Mark was at Vanderbilt staring at us blankly. Talking to Lucy was hard.

I remember our doctor came up to us in the hospital corridor on at least two occasions and said something like, "I'm afraid it's been too much; we're just not getting any response. I'm afraid it's been too much." He was not familiar with the drug she had taken and seemed to be having trouble finding out what else to do.

The thought that Lucy might not make it was intolerable to me. Mark came back to the hospital and stood beside me once, saying, "Mom, don't cry. You did all you could." I couldn't accept the hopelessness of his words and waved him away, saying, "No, no."

I can't remember what time it was when our doctor came out of the ICU with a wide grin and said, "She's awake! She's been talking to us!" He explained that another local doctor, familiar with drugs used in anesthesia, had given Lucy a medication that awakened her.

"I asked her how many of those pills she swallowed," Dr. Chaney continued, "and she started holding up fingers; we counted thirty-five. She's not out of the woods yet," he cautioned, "but this is a good sign."

A little while later he came back to tell us, "She's still responding. She wants a Big Mac and some french fries." Lucy had scrawled these barely legible words on a scrap of paper. I kept it for a long time, but it was finally lost.

While she was still in the ICU, my mind hurried ahead, wondering if, having been so close to death, some change in her brain's functioning might restore her mental balance. I thought this might be a first step back to real recovery, physically and mentally.

Lucy was awakened periodically and given the miracle drug that had brought her out of the coma until she began responding on her own and was taken off the respirator early the next day. She went back to Plateau on Sunday, May 23, with a good physical recovery from a nearly fatal act, but we saw no change mentally.

She was discharged from Plateau around the middle of June, and our lives went on almost normally. On August 12, a beautiful, cool day, I wrote, "Lucy is making macaroni and cheese for supper. She saw Dr. Johnson yesterday. She's done exercises, taken a bike ride and walk through the neighborhood yesterday, and is working on a Humpty Dumpty (cloth stuffed doll)."

Lucy seemed to be doing fairly well that summer, but Mark began suffering continuing periods of darkest depression. He preregistered for classes at the University of Tennessee, Knoxville in June and made a trip to Maryland with me in late August. Shortly before this trip, he overdosed on some vitamins and was kept overnight at the hospital after emergency room treatment. On September 16, he was back in the hospital after another, more serious overdose on some of Lucy's medicine. I don't remember what it was. His doctor told us that the mental confusion and physical symptoms (convulsive spasms that wracked his body) that he had at that time might be irreversible. These symptoms gradually subsided after anxious days, and he made a good recovery.

He still wanted to go to the University of Tennessee, Knoxville, and his doctor okayed his plans to start the fall term before discharging him from the hospital. We were not happy about his going, but we were so worn out from the summer's stress, we didn't try to hold him back. I know now that he was totally unfit for a college campus at that time.

On Saturday, September 25, Mark disappeared from his UT dormitory, and we made frantic efforts to locate him. I was certain that we had lost him, and we learned later that he had planned suicide. The crisis ended when we finally traced him to a motel and got him hospitalized in Knoxville.

Lucy was skipping her medicine. "I don't need any medicine," she said and adamantly refused to take it. She began staying in her room, talking to her calculator, and saying bizarre things that kept us on edge. Her condition worsened as September disappeared, and in October, we were faced with the hardest decision of our lives—forced commitment to a state hospital. One of my worst memories will always be her last departure from the farm in the back of a patrol car when two deputies drove her away without a word as Frank and I stood by.

Chapter Eight

OCTOBER 1982 – FEBRUARY 1984

A Widening Gap

Lucy gradually improved at the state hospital, Moccasin Bend Mental Health Institute, after our traumatic parting at the Cookeville jail.

She was cheerful, though still confused, when we first visited her in Chattanooga. We had no idea what a state mental hospital was like, and while it was depressing, as most state institutions are, we were glad to find a modern building with courtyards and sunny corridors. I was relieved that Lucy's hostility had gone, and she didn't seem to resent the part we had played in her forced hospitalization.

Frank and I were going back and forth between the private hospital in Knoxville to see Mark and Chattanooga to see Lucy that fall. During one of our visits to see Mark, we spoke to his psychiatrist about Lucy. We gave him a brief history of her illness and present situation, and I asked, "If she were your daughter, what would you do?"

"If she were my daughter, I'd try to get her into the National Institute of Mental Health," he replied. We were five years into our struggle with schizophrenia before we heard of this facility.

"What is that?" I asked. Dr. Carlton briefly described the federally funded research hospital that was then part of the National Institutes of Health in Bethesda, Maryland. He was familiar with a current schizophrenia research program at NIMH and he thought Lucy might qualify as a patient.

"She'll have to meet all the criteria for a diagnosis of chronic schizophrenia. She'll have to sign herself in voluntarily for treatment if she's accepted, and she may be there for six months or a year. As a patient of NIMH, all of her expenses there will be free, and there's a chance they may find the answer."

Frank and I found this information exciting and hopeful and asked when the arrangements could be made. "I'll need to make an evaluation of her condition here," he said, advising that Lucy could be transferred from Moccasin Bend to Parkwest Medical Center in Knoxville for a three-week period of observation. We were thrilled at this unexpected opportunity and glad that Lucy could leave the state hospital for a chance that seemed to be heaven-sent.

Everyone we talked with about the National Institute of Mental Health that fall thought it would be a wonderful opportunity for Lucy, and the best thing we could possibly do to help her. Her psychiatrist at Moccasin Bend was skeptical when we mentioned having Lucy transferred to a private hospital, but after we explained it was a prelude to going to NIMH, he agreed it was a great opportunity and filled out the papers for the transfer.

Lucy was delighted with the idea and signed release forms

so that all of her medical records, from the two psychiatrists we had consulted in Nashville and those from Plateau Mental Health Center and Moccasin Bend, could be forwarded to Dr. Carlton in Knoxville as quickly as possible.

Frank and I drove Lucy from Chattanooga to Knoxville the first week of November and saw her settled in at Parkwest, a brand-new, cheerful hospital with carpeted halls that contrasted sharply with Moccasin Bend. We were filled with more hope than we'd known since Lucy's first breakdown.

"If nothing else," Dr. Carlton said, "You'll know you have done everything possible—you'll have been to Mecca."

Lucy had a pleasant room for her short stay in the new hospital and seemed pleased, but she was still smiling one minute and tearful the next. One morning when we stopped to see her after visiting Mark, a nurse told us Lucy had done something unexpected.

"What happened?" I asked, instantly afraid she had done something to injure herself.

"It's not really serious," the nurse answered, "but she looks different than the last time you saw her."

Lucy came out of her room and down the hall to greet us about that time, and she looked strange indeed. Her eyebrows were gone. The nurse explained that she had asked for a razor to shave her legs but instead, she had shaved off her eyebrows.

"We'll be more careful from now on," she said. We were thankful it wasn't worse. Lucy did not want to talk about her reasons for doing this except to indicate it had improved her appearance.

The three weeks at Parkwest passed quickly. Lucy met all the requirements for a diagnosis of chronic schizophrenia that NIMH required, and Dr. Carlton made the arrangements for our appointment in Bethesda. We picked Lucy up at the hospital one morning the latter part of November and left Knoxville with high expectations for the drive to Maryland.

It was a tense, tiring drive, but Lucy napped a lot, and we were glad she was willing to make the journey. She was agreeable about taking her medicine, but we felt she was in a barely stable and highly unpredictable condition. We had no idea whether she would sign herself in for the program if she were accepted at NIMH, and no idea what we would do if she didn't.

We stopped overnight at a motel just outside Washington so we could have a meal and some rest before facing the whizzing traffic into Bethesda early the next morning. The huge complex of buildings that comprised the National Institutes of Health was pretty intimidating to all of us. We finally found the right building, a cavernous place full of bustling activity and hurrying people, and went to the floor where the professionals we were scheduled to see had their offices.

We met all of the staff members who would be working with Lucy, looked over the unit where she would be staying, and convened for a conference. Lucy didn't talk a lot, but Frank and I told the doctors and social worker present everything we could recall about her illness, including her attempted suicide in May of that year.

"It's just a miracle she's sitting here," I said. "If we hadn't been trying to get her up that morning to go to a day care program, she wouldn't be."

"Did you do that, Lucy?" a doctor asked.

Lucy answered without hesitation, "Yes, but I had to do it." She might have been talking about drinking a soda or something equally innocuous.

All of the research procedures were explained to Lucy and to us; we were shown around the building, ate lunch in the large, crowded cafeteria, and returned to our floor for more consultations.

I can't remember the details of the research Lucy was to take part in, but we knew it would not be easy for her and would require a lot of patience on her part. Our overall impression was that she would still have the most individual treatment and evaluation that we could hope for, and we were favorably impressed with all the staff. As I recall, there were only about ten or eleven patients in the unit, and I thought something good would surely come from such a closely monitored period of research, treatment, and therapy.

During the course of our talks with the doctors at NIMH that day, one of the psychiatrists said, "You need to understand there is no guarantee that we'll be able to find the answer here. It may be necessary for Lucy to go from this hospital to some other one." His words flitted through my mind and returned like a dark shadow. Why would she need to go to some other hospital? If she didn't get better here, she would surely just go home again. She would be an outpatient at Plateau as before, but another hospital? The shadow hovered only momentarily. In that busy place that supported some of the finest research minds in the country, there was too much hope in our hearts to think of anything but vast improvement.

Relief flooded through us like a shot of adrenaline when Lucy agreed to sign herself in sometime during the afternoon. We met her roommate, saw her room, and left in the late afternoon, feeling that she was in good hands.

"We'll call you as soon as we get home, Luce," we told her, waving a last good-bye to her on the locked unit that would be her residence for several months. Lucy seemed satisfied for the moment with her new surroundings and had washed her hair and rolled it up while we were still conferring with the doctors. As I remember, her unit had a sitting room, a corridor of bedrooms with gray, metal beds, and facilities for cooking and eating.

Lucy's months at NIMH, from November 1982 until May 1983, passed quickly and were filled with strain at home. Mark's behavior had become increasingly unpredictable. His condition was diagnosed as a manic-depressive illness in January 1983, when he was again hospitalized in Knoxville, this time at Lakeshore Mental Health Institution, the state hospital there. We were thankful Lucy wasn't at home that winter. We felt comforted to think that she, at least, was getting the best possible treatment at the time, and we hoped that NIMH might come up with a real breakthrough for her.

It was impossible for us to participate in her treatment in person as the hospital would have liked, but we were in touch weekly by telephone and were very thankful for the close contact. We mailed her a box of Christmas gifts in December, but the package was either stolen or lost in the mail. Lucy was very disappointed, and I was disgusted with the U.S. postal service. Frank had to make a trip to Washington in January, and we tried to duplicate all of the lost gifts and sent them with him to deliver in person. He had a short visit with Lucy at the hospital, and she was pleased with her presents.

During the latter part of January, February, and March of that year, Lucy had periods of being unable to talk to us over the phone. Sometimes she would scream and demand that we come and pick her up that instant. When we tried to explain why this was not possible, she would shriek until one of the nurses or her social worker came to the phone.

"We can't let Lucy talk when she's like this, Mrs. Holloway. It doesn't do her any good, and I'm sure it doesn't do you all any good."

We knew Lucy was having bad times, and we worried, but there was nothing we could do from such a distance. The social worker explained that sometimes patients were put in wet sheets when they became extremely agitated. "It may sound cruel, but it has a calming effect on a person in that state, and sometimes it's the only thing that helps." We were told on at least two occasions when we called to ask about her that Lucy had "been in sheets."

We decided to sell our ten acres on the mountain and move to town that winter. I told Lucy of the change over the telephone, and she seemed glad about the move to town but a little sad too. Selling our animals and leaving the country was hard for me, but it had all become too much for us to manage. The house we purchased was near Frank's work at the university, and we thought it would be ideal for Lucy. She had never liked being "way out here" during our years at the farm.

We had moved a number of times, but the move to Cookeville in April 1983 was the hardest I can remember. We were just getting settled when NIMH called to say that Lucy would be discharged from the hospital in May. In order to participate in research, she had been taken off of all antipsychotic drugs. Without the medicine, Lucy became extremely psychotic and out-of-control, and they could not continue with her in the research program for that reason.

We were extremely disappointed by this news, but one of our questions had been answered. We had always wondered what would happen if Lucy were taken off the drugs. We hated the medicine as much as she did and had hoped that someday she could be free of it. The answer from NIMH was not cheering.

We made the 1,200-mile round-trip to Bethesda to bring Lucy home the first part of May. We visited briefly with the nurses and Lucy's social worker. Lucy said her good-byes to some of the patients, obviously happy to be leaving the hospital, and we were glad she was coming home.

The main thing we learned from Lucy's six months at NIMH was that she would have to remain on antipsychotic drugs in order to maintain any stability. We were told that she was cooperative with the research procedures that she took part in there, but we never had any detailed conversation with anyone at NIMH about her behavior when she was off the drugs or anything else regarding her stay there. We were disappointed not to have learned more, but I will always remember the kindness and understanding of the nurses and social worker who worked with Lucy in that hospital.

When I started writing this book in 1984, I wrote to Lucy's social worker at NIMH and asked if she or any of the nurses there who knew Lucy could tell me their impressions of Lucy and anything about her during the time she was there. Lucy's social worker replied as follows: "I can only say that I know that while Lucy was here, she had some good times and some very rough times. I would have to say that her main strength is her ability to get people interested in her, and her sweetness, when she is not so frightened by her own inner turmoil. She has a childlike quality that engages other people. Also, this childlike quality will not be helpful to her when she grows a bit older. As you know, one of her difficulties is her stubbornness (or apparent stubbornness) when she wants to do something. Considering the nature of this hospitalization and the difficulty with the research, she did very well here. I look forward to talking to you at some point and add my hopes to yours that Lucy makes some gains."

Along with her letter, she sent me the name of a support group for families, Families in Touch, in Nashville, which was the beginning of our acquaintance with the National Alliance for the Mentally Ill (NAMI), and a movement that remains important in our lives.

A lot of things were going on at home that spring when Lucy returned and began making the painful transition from the hospital back to the real world. Her older brother was in Johnson City,

Tennessee, looking for a job and planning to be married in June. Mark had been discharged from Lake Shore Mental Health Institution in Knoxville in February and was working temporarily at a furniture company. My husband was scheduled to have major surgery in June, and our future daughter-in-law was graduating from Tennessee Tech University that same month.

Lucy's first few weeks at home went well. She took her medicine without protest, took walks around the new neighborhood, and planned to attend a day care program at Plateau, which had been recommended by NIMH. My journal for May 30, reads, "Lucy fixed a delicious tuna casserole supper with bran muffins and helped put up about eight pints of strawberries we picked yesterday at the farm." (We still owned the farm at that time). She and Frank and I got them picked just before it rained."

In early June, Lucy began withdrawing and staying in her room more. On June 8, she was back at Plateau to see her doctor, and signed in as an inpatient at her own request. She was there for two weeks and came home on June 18. I found a note, "Lucy home from Plateau. Not doing well. Depressed."

The spring and summer of 1983 passed too quickly, and Lucy's continuing problems with depression, withdrawal, and unpredictable actions brought strain, frustration, and often anger to all of us. Sometime during that summer, Frank and I realized that one of us would have to stay with Lucy at all times. We were afraid to trust leaving her alone anymore.

I thought that having some regular chores to do at home would help, and I assigned tasks. "I want you to vacuum upstairs and clean the bathroom. Would you like to cook dinner one night a week?"

Lucy responded enthusiastically to these suggestions ("I'd love to!") but it never lasted. Now I know that the turmoil in her mind must have made it almost impossible for her to concentrate. I told Frank one day, "Maybe if she could do the shopping, handle the money, and make out the grocery lists, she'd get interested and better at it." I thought it would help her to get out and learn to buy the groceries and cook again. I thought she was going to get better and just needed a little help getting started.

Frank took her shopping one morning, but apparently it was a sporadic, stressful trip for him with Lucy going off in all directions, putting things into the cart without thinking. When they returned, he told me, "You take her next time. I'll not try it again," weariness in every syllable.

One afternoon Lucy gathered all of her old textbooks from Tennessee Tech in her room, saying, "I'm going to review these for when I start back to school."

I knew she wasn't ready to handle university work then, and told her, "You can't plan on that right now, Luce. Maybe later."

We knew she wasn't well enough to undertake most of the things she wanted to do that summer, and "maybe later" became a melancholy refrain. I remember the frustrating conversations we had.

"When are we going back to InterVarsity?"

"They aren't having it this summer, Luce. Maybe we can go later."

"I've decided I just want to get a job and work. I don't want to go to day care anymore. I want to be on my own."

"Lucy, you need to try day care for a while. Maybe later we can see about a job."

"Can I take driving lessons again? I already know how to drive; all I need is a little brushing up."

"Not now, Lucy. Maybe later."

In early August, after continuing problems with depression, she went back to Plateau for a period of about three weeks. When she returned, Mark was preparing to try another term at the University of Tennessee in Knoxville, and Lucy said, "I want to take some classes at Tech this fall."

"You're not ready for that yet. You need to try day care for a while longer," I told her. "We'll see about Tech later."

With growing frustration, she answered, "I want to live in my own place—please! (whining) I just want to get a job and have my own place then. It's not fair. I need to be on my own."

"Lucy, you just aren't ready yet. You've got to accept it. Maybe later…"

I wonder now how many times I yelled at her when the tears and suicide threats, the whining and the constant mood swings made me frantic. I wonder now if Lucy was slowly absorbing all those negative messages: no more InterVarsity fellowship, no more Tech, no more learning to drive, no more plans about getting a job, no more hope of having a room or apartment of her own…

Several times she locked herself in the upstairs bathroom,

shrieking, "I want to kill myself!" running the water full blast with a roar that turned my heart to jelly. I pounded up the stairs, yelling, "Lucy, Lucy! Turn off that water and open the door now! Open the door this minute!" She always opened the door eventually, but the strain of those moments lingered for days.

I remember other peaceful days when Lucy went to bed early and scolded me for coming up later to tuck her in. "Mom, I can do that. I'm not a baby!" We were always thankful when she could sleep and enjoy a television show or a walk or any normal activity.

Frankie and Ruth came home for a visit in October and Lucy inexplicably chopped off all of her hair with a razor blade. Her reason for doing it was similar to the one she gave when she had shaved off her eyebrows at Parkwest. She said it looked better. She had cut it so short that we bought a wig. She wore it a number of times, but it never looked natural and the effect was worse than the butchered hair.

All during October, Lucy suffered depression daily and was often in tears. She couldn't seem to concentrate on anything for long. She was eating enormous amounts of food at home, and at one point she told her doctor at Plateau that she had been raped. She was questioned and examined about this story, and her doctor assured us it wasn't true. Later, Lucy said she had made it up, but her reason for eating so much was that she was pregnant.

On October 31, I wrote, "Lucy spent all weekend inside, mostly in her room. She didn't have as many violent mood swings as last week but just doesn't seem to want to do anything."

Her continuing cycles of depression, tears, and constant frustration seemed to be building toward a dreaded climax.

Chapter Nine

NOVEMBER 1983 – MARCH 1984

"I Don't Want To Live"

All of our remaining hopes from the National Institute of Mental Health had faded by the fall of 1983. The new house and the new beginnings we'd thought of—Lucy getting involved in some activities, making new friends, learning a craft or hobby—just never happened.

She withdrew from us more and more.

"Play badminton with me, Luce."

"Not now. I want to read."

"Come for a walk, Lucy."

"Later, I'm reading now." (closed in her room)

"Do you want to go shopping, Luce?"

"Not now. I want to lose some weight first."

On the morning of November 25 she overdosed on a small amount of Stelazine (antipsychotic drug) and some complexion medicine she had found. She had been very restless, depressed, and troubled with voices (hearing voices) for several days. Frank and I woke up sometime around four o'clock that morning when we heard her walking around the house. "Lucy, what are you doing?" I called, and she opened our door and told us of the overdose.

Frank pulled on some clothes and rushed her to the emergency room of Cookeville General. She was given something like charcoal to trap the drugs and induce vomiting. Frank stayed at the hospital until about 7:30 that morning when she seemed fairly stable. She was admitted for observation to be sure there was no kidney or liver damage and taken to a room on the third floor. She seemed physically okay by the following day, and we took her to Plateau for what we thought would be a few more days of observation and rest.

She came home for a weekend leave on December 1, and I wrote, "Lucy home for weekend. She and Frank went to church and took a gift for needy families. Lucy stayed very active yesterday; walked, watched television some and played checkers and games with Mark for short periods. Seems better though still troubled with voices and lack of concentration. She bought new jeans and blouse yesterday when she went shopping with Frank."

I had no idea what Lucy was thinking or feeling deep down in that part of her mind that we could only catch glimpses of then. The enormity of her problems washed over me in waves of sadness at times. Her days at home went by so fast, all cluttered with cooking and cleaning and running here and there, and then, after she went back to Plateau, there was a silence. I slowly realized that something precious had been there, but it had slipped away. It had slipped away during all those rushing months from May till November when we were still settling in, going to Ruthie's graduation, waiting through Frank's surgery, sharing Frankie and Ruth's marriage…

During December Lucy told us, "Dr. Davis (her new psychiatrist at Plateau) thinks I have a chronic illness, but it's really my arrogance. That's my whole illness; I'm just too arrogant." And she wrote a prayer, "Dear Lord Jesus, please help me to think of others as better than myself, to realize I'm not worthy, Dear Lord Jesus..."

She came home for a four-day Christmas leave from Plateau. I remember how she comforted me one day when she caught me crying because of her condition. "Don't cry, Mom! There, there, don't cry," she said, enveloping me in a huge hug. "You're the kindest, wisest, most wonderful mother in the world—don't cry!"

She tried to give away all of her Christmas gifts that year because "I don't deserve them." Frankie and Ruth gave her a sketch pad and water colors and Frankie tried to interest her in them, but she walked away up to her room. Sometime later she sketched a clown face on the pad. I found it on her bed after she went back to Plateau.

Something had slipped away in the clatter of dishes and laughter at the Christmas table at Ruthie's house. I still see Lucy's blank expression, her lost, silent, depressed look while plates were passed and quips exchanged and music blared from a tape of old songs from the forties and fifties when some of us were young.

I remember the Christmas cards she asked for. Frank bought her a new box after she rejected the ones I gave her and insisted on new ones. Later, we found she had torn them up, and I scolded, "Lucy, did you tear up the whole box? Why did you tear them up? Don't ask us to buy any more. Those were expensive cards."

I didn't know then that she couldn't write them. I looked at the pieces later, torn scraps of salutations and beginnings scrawling into nothingness, unfinished notes written over and over…And I knew why her ears were deaf to quarreling protests about wasted money or torn cards. Something infinitely more valuable had been wasted. Something that was Lucy had been wasted and lost and cut into pieces like the scrawled notes. Something that was Lucy had slipped away…

After Christmas, things continued to go downhill for Lucy at Plateau. Dr. Davis tried different medicines, but none seemed to bring any lasting stability. The self-destructive acts continued. She darted into the dining hall and blistered her mouth with scalding coffee one day. She burned her hand with hot water—"for punishment." Frank and I looked at her reddened hand later and asked, "Was it an accident, Luce?"

"No."

"You did it on *purpose?*"

"Yes, yes." She looked at us quickly. "It's all right. Stop looking at me like that."

On January 7, 1984, I wrote, "Went to bed in prayer and at peace. Woke in tears thinking of Lucy as we saw her last night. She is some better. Some of the heavy breathing and agitation is quieter. They (Plateau staff) said she had 'slept some,' had 'eaten some.' There were dark circles under her eyes, but she came walking out to see us with that eager, plunging gait…"

One evening, the nurse told us she was too upset for any

company. "Everything that's in her head is coming out of her mouth right now," was the way she put it.

On another day in January we brought her a milkshake. We sat before the sterile, artificial fire in the "blue room" at Plateau and tried to visit. Lucy's periods of concentration were very brief. She seemed uninterested in drinking the milkshake; she just stared blankly and held it. Her eyes blinked rapidly at intervals and she rocked back and forth and chanted to herself over and over. I made out some of the words. "Push, young lady, push, young lady, push young lady. Honey chile, you'd better talk, young lady, push young lady, honey chile, young lady..."

"You'd better drink that shake, honey chile," I said, hoping to break up the chanting. Lucy looked up quickly and smiled for a moment.

"All right," she said, and took a big swallow. "Mom, I love you. Dad, thank you for this milkshake." She finished up the last of it and lapsed into silence. Between lost, mute periods she asked, "How is Heidi?" (dog) "How is Max?" (cat) Her smile came suddenly for seconds, that wonderful, all-enveloping childlike smile that lights up her face like a million candles.

"What have you all been doing?" she asked suddenly, and I told her of washing clothes, cleaning house, of missing her, and of some friends who had asked about her. She smiled briefly. "Uh-huh. That's nice." Then she was back to chanting and rocking. Finally, there were good-bye hugs.

"We'll see you tomorrow. Drink your juice. Try to sleep."

"I love you, Mom—Dad."

"Love you too, Luce, love you too..."

What was the most overpoweringly sad thing to me then was the thought, since talking to her doctor that week, that the past Christmas would be the last one Lucy would have at home for a long time, and that she knew it. Equally overpowering was my terrible fear that she would come home, and we would go back to being caretakers and medicine dispensers, under the constant strain of wondering what she would do next.

I remembered her last days at home when we were afraid to leave her alone for any length of time. I thought of the times we had wondered anxiously what she was doing up in her room as we listened to the sounds of drawers being jerked open, furniture moved, endless steps. I thought of her lying in her disheveled bed, half undressed, saying so many times, "I want to rest. I want to take a nap. I'm reading," as she closed the door and shut us out.

On January 10 my journal reads, "Lucy got a burn equivalent to sunburn when she jumped into hot shower. Dr. Davis told us it was mostly on her stomach and upper thighs." When we visited her the last week in January, she was very tearful and depressed and told us, "I don't want to live."

On another visit we saw that she was having a lot of trouble with voices. She rocked back and forth, blinked rapidly, and said sadly once, "I never know what to say to people." We told her it didn't matter, that most people talk too much, but I don't think it comforted her.

Frank, trying to make conversation, looked across the courtyard to another unit where some patients were sitting around a table and said, "I see a whole bunch of people sitting at a table over there, Lucy."

"Yes," she said. "They're playing cards."

"Do you play cards, Luce?" I asked.

She looked at me for a long, lucid moment and said, "No, Mama." Something about her tone made me feel she meant that was something she might never be doing again. When we left, she took our hands and prayed, as she sometimes does, "Dear Lord, keep my parents safe on the way home. Amen."

We saw little change in Lucy when the cold, gray days of February came. Dr. Davis was not optimistic when we spoke to him about her. "Lucy is one of the sickest patients I've ever treated," he said once. On February 8, Lucy called Frank a number of times at work and also called me at home. She was very agitated and tearful and asked me once, "Mom, what's wrong with me?" Once she asked Frank, "Dad, what's ever going to become of me?"

Nothing has ever torn our hearts as much as those sad, searching questions that we couldn't answer. Dr. Davis told us, "She talks of being electrocuted for bad things she thinks she has done." She confessed all sorts of crimes to us too, and said again during a visit, "I don't want to live because my head is all messed up."

When we visited her on Thursday, February 23, we thought she seemed a little better. She was very sweet and affectionate with us, but her lucid moments came and went constantly. She clung to us, held our hands, and several times looked into my face as if trying to see into my very soul. I felt she was desperately trying to hang on to some kind of control, but she was constantly responding audibly to voices. Just before we left, she said, "I have something for you."

She ran back to her unit and returned with two oval flower prints, suitable for decoupage, that she had cut out. "Do you like them?" she asked. I told her I did and could use them for wall plaques. She looked pleased for a moment.

When we spoke to Dr. Davis about this visit later, I was shocked when he told us that, just before we came, Lucy had accused a male staff member of touching her breast and had hit him "as hard as she could."

The next day, February 24, Dr. Davis called to say that he was having Lucy transported to Moccasin Bend because they could not control her behavior at Plateau any longer. While he was talking with me about her, someone told him that Lucy had dashed into the dining hall and scalded her mouth with hot coffee again. As I recall it, Dr. Davis left the phone and went to examine her. He called back to tell me he was sending her on to Chattanooga since he didn't think the burn was serious, and that it would probably heal in a day or two.

Somewhere around 8:30 a.m. on February 25, a supervising nurse at Moccasin Bend telephoned us to say that they had taken Lucy to Baroness Erlanger Hospital in Chattanooga because they were very concerned about her burned throat and lips, the breathing difficulty she was having, and the swelling and obvious infection she was suffering from.

"Someone was observing her all night here," the nurse said, "but I was really shocked at her condition when I came in this morning." She asked me about Lucy's treatment at Plateau and why they had sent her in that condition. I told her the doctor in charge had apparently failed to recognize the seriousness of the burn. My mind was filled with pictures of Lucy being driven to the Bend with her burned mouth, spending the long night there in pain, with nobody who loved her nearby.

Frank and I drove to Chattanooga that morning. Nothing could have prepared us for Lucy's appearance. She held up her arms and tried to kiss us with her horribly swollen mouth when we came into the hospital room. They were giving her IVs and antibiotics for the infection, which the doctor treating her said was very bad.

We were impressed with the care she was getting, but her condition stunned us. The nurses told us it would be better if we didn't go in to see her too often because she tried to talk whenever she saw us. We stayed on the hospital ward until late afternoon, looking in on her at intervals, and decided to stay overnight in the hotel that was part of the hospital. After a meal in the hospital dining room, we fell into bed, thankful to be near Lucy, totally exhausted.

By Sunday afternoon, the outside of her mouth had healed a lot, but she was still on IVs and antibiotics. The nurse told us there was nothing we could do by staying, so we drove back to Cookeville after telling Lucy good-bye. She seemed pretty calm, and we thought she might stay quieter if we weren't there.

She was later moved to the psychiatric wing of Erlanger, where nurses reported she was healing rapidly and doing well. She telephoned us several times on Monday, February 27, but it was hard to understand what she said. Her voice still sounded bubbly and she was apparently very confused.

When I called Erlanger on Thursday to ask about her, a nurse said, "Darling, they took her back to the Bend today." I was disappointed that they hadn't kept her longer in that beautiful, efficient hospital, but the nurse assured me that she was recovering well and her throat was no longer infected. I telephoned Moccasin Bend but was told I couldn't talk to Lucy yet, to call back in a day or two. We planned to drive down on Saturday anyway, so I resigned myself to wait.

On Friday a friend went with me to Plateau to see Dr. Davis and to pick up Lucy's things that were still there. Dr. Davis was very sorry about what had happened. I felt he would never have sent her if he had realized how seriously she was burned.

I didn't know how much it would hurt seeing her belongings at Plateau—her battered pocketbook, her clothes, two Bibles she always wanted with her, and a little tile trivet she had made in crafts. I knew she wouldn't be coming back to Plateau in the foreseeable future, and it was as if she had died.

Saturday, March 3, was a beautiful spring day for our trip to Moccasin Bend. We knew Lucy could not be too well, but Frank and I had to hold back tears when we saw her. She walked into the visiting area wearing a hospital robe, pajamas, and slippers, hair uncombed, pale, shaky, and vacant-eyed. She was almost totally incoherent at first, but then she said, "Hi, Mama," and came into my arms. She held on for a long moment in silence. Then she kissed Frank and held on to him. Her old smile was gone and her eyes seemed far away, but she seemed to be very aware of what was going on. She said, "I want to talk to you," and "I love you," several times and then just held us in silence again.

Frank sat with her while I tried to get some information from the nurse about her condition. "She's getting on all right," she told me. "The infection is gone, but she's still very weak."

We could see Lucy was very tired and told her we were going on back to Cookeville so she could rest. "Mom, what's been going on?" she asked. I explained what had happened and told her she would soon be better. "Are you staying in the hotel?" she asked, and I guess she was thinking of the hotel at Erlanger. She seemed tired to the point of passing out, and we tried not to talk anymore. Finally she said, "I'm tired," and we watched her stumble back to the unit with the help of a technician.

She was better, though still weak, when we visited her on March 10. The best thing was her smile when we came in. Most of her conversation was in touch with reality, but when Frank left to get her a soda from the lobby, she said loudly, "I am the fallen angel."

"No, you're just Lucy Holloway," I said. She accepted it.

"Am I Satan?" she asked a moment later.

"No. You're just Lucy. You're a good person, Luce. You always have been. I'm your mama, so I should know, shouldn't I?"

She looked at me intently for a moment with a strange light in her eyes and said, "Mama, you have the prettiest eyes!"

"Well, you still have that million-dollar smile," I said. She looked pleased and asked, "I have?" But her smile was not quite the same. Something had changed that I couldn't put my finger on.

When we went home, all I could think of was Lucy, remembering happier days. I thought of the times at the farm when she had wanted me to listen to her favorite James Taylor and Anne Murray records. Music was important to her then. We had walked around the basement with books on our heads for posture and danced to Tony Orlando and Dawn, giggling and singing along with "Say Has Anybody Seen My Sweet Gypsy Rose," "Knock Three Times," and "Who's In The Strawberry Patch With Sally." It was another part of Lucy that seemed to be gone, one more loss that weighed on my heart like a stone.

It was a beautiful, crisp, sunny day when Mark, Frank, and I drove to Chattanooga for Lucy's twenty-third birthday. We brought along a chocolate cake, a pink stuffed bunny, a small lace pillow for her room, and a poster from Mark. I also had a new T-shirt and cotton duster that I hoped she would like.

Lucy met us with a smile and a hug, but the visit was sketchy. Frank and I tried to talk with the supervising nurse a few minutes while Mark stayed with Lucy and brought her an orange soda from the lobby. She was always thirsty because of the medicine.

While we were talking in an adjoining office, the nurse paused and listened for a moment. "I hear singing," she said. She stepped into the hall and returned to tell us, "Yes, that's your children singing out there, and it's a very good sign for Lucy, the first time she's done anything like that."

When we went back to the visitor's room, they were sitting at an old piano there. Mark had picked out some Beatles and Billy Joel songs on the ancient instrument that Lucy remembered. It made us happy seeing them that way.

Later, Lucy ate some of the gooey cake, put on her new duster, and seemed pleased with the other gifts. Suddenly, apparently responding to some hallucination, her eyes lost contact, and she struck out at the nurse who was laughing and talking to her about the gifts.

A male attendant came over, and Lucy struck out at him too. The visit ended abruptly as they led her, protesting loudly, back to the unit. Another staff member told us, "She'll be okay in a little while."

"No, she won't be okay," I thought. "Not okay at all."

Chapter Nine
SUMMER 1988

Moccasin Bend

It will soon be five years since Lucy went to the state hospital for the second time on that bleak February day in 1984. She did not go gently into her night of isolation and exile from the world. She went crying and shrieking, clutching the last remnants of her normalcy with frightened, frantic hands, doing violence to herself with increasing severity. We tried to visit her every week for a long time, but now we go every other week.

During the early spring of 1984 I wrote several long letters to staff members, detailing things we hoped Lucy might be helped to do, telling them what she had liked and had been able to do before schizophrenia. I sent them an eleven-page chronology of her illness from 1978 to 1984, thinking we would discuss it at some point. Nobody ever referred to those letters or discussed anything regarding them with us at that time or in the years since.

One very intelligent and understanding woman, who was then director of Nursing Education at Moccasin Bend, was more helpful. A nurse on Lucy's unit introduced us to Mrs. Roland one day while we were visiting Lucy. She explained that part of her job was working with families if that was desired. "If you like," she told us, "I can visit with Lucy every week and then talk with you about things I feel might be helpful for her recovery."

That someone in the hospital would be having that kind of one-on-one contact with Lucy every week and would talk to us about whatever insights she gained was the answer to my prayers. We were elated at a chance to work actively with someone from the hospital who seemed optimistic about Lucy's chances for recovery.

As it turned out, we never had any of the conferences we were looking forward to so eagerly that summer. Mrs. Roland became ill in July and had to resign her position at the hospital. We never heard anymore about this kind of relationship between Moccasin Bend staff and a family, and we were very disappointed.

Our attempts to learn what was going on with Lucy were usually hurried conversations with a technician, nurse, or social worker when we visited the hospital. We learned little from the scattered conferences we had with her doctor of the moment and nothing about any consistent plan of treatment.

Lucy was often in tears that year, and she couldn't understand why we didn't take her home. Once, when she was having a lot of trouble putting words together, she muttered fiercely, "I can't think, I can't even think!" On another visit she told us, "I want to have a long talk without the voices," a poignant hope that still seems tragically impossible. She is usually mumbling to voices whenever we visit.

Since she is unable to communicate coherently much of the time, we don't really know what experiences Lucy has had in the hospital. She was moved from unit to unit in the main building during 1984 and early 1985. Each move resulted in great confusion and agitation for her and frustration for us as we tried to find out who her new doctor, social worker, and other staff members were and what had happened to her continually disappearing clothes. The problem with her clothes remains unsolved to this day, a chronic fact of life in the hospital.

We weren't usually informed when Lucy was being moved, but I got a telephone call from Lucy's social worker on March 12, 1985, advising that they were moving her to the Winston Building, the long-term care facility, the next day. We had earlier requested that she be put on the waiting list for Winston Building, but we were unprepared for its overcrowded, understaffed units. Some members of the Tennessee legislature seemed to be hell-bent on closing down beds at Moccasin Bend that year, even though there was no place for the patients in many of those beds to go.

We waited until Friday of the next week to visit Lucy. It was her twenty-fourth birthday, and we hoped she might be more adjusted to the move by that time.

Noise and confusion greeted us when we stepped through the door of her unit that March day. A wall-mounted television blared, a stereo pounded, and a cacophony of voices babbled in our ears. The atmosphere bordered on chaos. Lucy came running to meet us from her wing of the unit, and I went down the hall with a nurse to see if her clothes had been brought over from the main building. We couldn't find anything that belonged to Lucy. She had been at Winston Building for almost ten days, but none of her things were there.

We had brought Lucy a basket of treats and some gifts, and we went down to the lobby so she could eat the McDonald's dinner Frank had picked up. She unwrapped her presents there and Frank and I started to sing "Happy Birthday," but we couldn't make it. The words died away in painful silence.

Lucy talked to voices a lot during the visit and seemed to be totally confused, frustrated, and miserable. Finally, when we were back in her unit getting ready to leave, she stalked from us furiously, screaming, "I'll never get out of here! This place is awful!"

Lucy went back to her room, and I collapsed in tears of frustration and grief. I felt we should do something to change her situation, but I knew we couldn't take care of her at home. The cost of private care was out of the question. The social worker asked us to walk down the hall to an office where we could talk.

"It always takes at least three weeks for patients to adjust to a move," she told us. "She'll be a lot different the next time you see her. You and your husband need to stop worrying and get some rest. We'll take good care of her," she assured us later as we left the unit without seeing Lucy again.

My journal for March 24 reads, "Ever since we saw Lucy on Friday, have been haunted and depressed by the memory of her locked away on Unit B. My first impression of Unit B was—bedlam. Even after reassuring talk with social worker, doctor, and head nurse, I don't feel much better. Will call the hospital later today."

On a warm, breezy June day in 1986, we had a calmer visit. We sat in the bright, windowed lobby in the black, wrought iron chairs while Lucy drank a grape soda from the drink machine. She was all little-girl sweetness that day. There were no whining, guttural tones.

Suddenly, she laughed and said, "Show me some of Tom Barkley's guts!" It was a line Frank used to quote a lot from the TV series *The Big Valley*. Then she reached for my hand and said, "Let's all sing." She started "Row, row, row your boat," and I sang along for one squeaky chorus of the old round we used to sing when she and her brothers were little.

"Dad, let's waltz," she said as soon as the song ended. She pulled Frank to his feet, and they made a few turns but he protested, "I can't keep the beat."

We sat for a while longer and spoke to a patient who wanted some of Lucy's drink. Lucy started to give her the can, but I waved my hand and said, "Don't ever drink after anybody."

"Lucy may have germs. You don't want to get them, do you?" Frank asked the girl.

She smiled and said, "No." Then she added, still lingering beside us, "Just save me what you don't want, Lucy."

Frank bought her a soda too, and she walked away, still smiling.

It was a beautiful day, and we decided to take a walk around the building. Lucy looked pale, but her hair shone clean and coppery colored in the sun, and her thinner figure (she had been put on a diet) looked graceful in a pink, cotton skirt we'd brought her earlier. She wore an aqua blouse that looked pretty with her eyes.

"Let's sit on the porch," I suggested after we finished a short walk. We found places on a concrete patio outside the dining hall of the building and sat in the metal patio chairs holding hands. Sometimes Lucy leaned her head on my shoulder and I wondered what she was thinking.

"Let me give you a manicure," I told her, noticing several long, jagged nails. She sat quietly while I filed her nails, one of the few things I can do for her when we visit. I was glad she wasn't into voices much that day.

Once she said, "I can be a good girl, Dad." She hugged him close, planting kisses on his cheeks. Frank's eyes looked teary.

I thought how pretty she looked, how young and sweet, and I wished we could really talk. "Did you get my letter, Luce, with the chewing gum in it?" I asked.

"Yes, I got it," she answered, like a well-instructed little girl. She smiled suddenly. "Mom, you're the sweetest Mom in all the world," she said and hugged me.

"Let's walk back and look at the corn," Frank said, speaking of a small garden behind the building that we had seen on our last visit. The air was muggy and the sun had gotten hot, but we slid out of the chairs and walked toward the back.

"That corn needs weeding," Lucy said, looking at the dehydrated patch, which was being taken over by rampant weeds.

"That's too many weeds to think about," I said, feeling weary at the idea.

"I'd love to weed that garden," Lucy said brightly, and I remembered our years at the farm when she helped Frank weeding and pulling beans. I thought of the quart jars of tomato juice she had helped us can on Melrose Drive, and the last time she had helped Frank make jam from our own blackberries.

Back in the unit, we sat in the dayroom (between the male and female wings of the unit) while Lucy drank a last diet cola. She was still in good spirits and I was thankful. Finally, we said good-bye and Lucy stood at the door, looking out the glass pane while a nurse locked it, calling, "Good-bye, Mom and Dad! Thank you for coming to see me!"

I managed to keep back a flood of tears until we were out of sight. She had become too acclimated to the hospital, too accepting of its restrictions and frustrations, too "institutionalized." All her passionate pleas of earlier visits when she was first hospitalized—"I can't stand it here!" "I need to go home. Please! I'll never get well in this place!" "I need a weekend leave, please!"—had been missing for how long? Months? Years? Could three years have passed since she was home? It made me unbearably sad, and I saw it was the same for Frank.

The illness and the patients don't seem to have changed a lot in the almost forty years since I first looked at some pictures of mental patients in an old *LIFE* magazine, years before I was the wife and mother in a family or dreamed that such horror could touch one of my children.

We haven't seen any basic change in Lucy's condition in the four years she's been at the state hospital. No matter how much medicine she takes, the demons and delusions and the voices don't go away. Psychiatrists speak of a "rule of thirds" regarding the victims of schizophrenia. They have found that a third will recover, a third will improve and can function with help and proper medicine, and a third will not improve or recover. As of this writing, Lucy seems to be in that last third. We believe, if enough effort is made, research can find the answer to this disease within the next decade.

The care of patients like Lucy has a very low priority in our society. We know that the state hospital is chronically short of staff and that because of this, patients cannot get the quality of care that we would like.

This past March Lucy spent her twenty-seventh birthday on Unit A, Winston Building. Unit A is a locked unit for some of the poorest functioning patients.

Lucy walks with a shuffle now, and she is often lethargic and dull-eyed because of the large dose of antipsychotic drugs she takes. We worry about the long-term effect the drugs will have on her physically, and we wonder always what will become of her when we are gone.

When her medicine is reduced, as it has been at different times by different doctors, we are told, "Lucy gets wild; she runs, she screams, she takes her clothes off, she is seductive around male patients, she is a danger to herself, she disturbs others…" We know these things are true, but it's never easy to hear the words.

Somewhere in the cacophony and confusion, in the lost hopes and scattered dreams, somewhere in the unbelievable turmoil that is her mind, in that sometimes manipulative, demanding, screaming, sorrowing, frightened, whining, cajoling, sweet, affectionate little-girl woman is the daughter we have lost. She tried so hard to beat this illness; tried so hard, wrote so many prayers, made so many new resolutions, started back so gallantly from so many breakdowns...

The 200-mile-round trip we have to make every time we see our daughter gets harder every year. For now, the hospital doesn't think she is ready for weekend leaves at this distance, but telling her she can't come home is the hardest part of every visit.

In the spring of 1989 Lucy had several weekend leaves home. She has gradually gained and is maintaining a degree of stability that we didn't think possible at one time.

We hope this is only the beginning of better things...

Epilogue

SPRING 1989 – SPRING 1998

At the end of the book we published in 1989, I wrote that Lucy had had several weekend leaves home and we hoped this was the beginning of better things. She began coming home for visits that spring; but in March she suffered a second attack of Bell's palsy, a paralysis of the muscles of one side of the face, and was taken to Baroness Erlanger Hospital for treatment.

When we visited her in April, she had a patch over her left eye, her mouth was drawn down, and she had trouble with balance and in judging distance. She gradually recovered from the palsy (90 percent of patients do) and was able to come home for Mother's Day in May.

The next several months went well when Lucy came home for visits. She also enjoyed going to Hamilton Place and Eastgate malls in Chattanooga when we visited her. She had a Thanksgiving visit home that year, but on December 10, we learned that lab work, verified at Erlanger Hospital, showed "abnormal kidney function." She was taken off the antipsychotic drugs she had been on and was put on a very restricted, low-salt diet. Despite our efforts to learn the exact cause of her condition and the extent of the damage, we never got definitive answers. I had anxious visions of her having to go on dialysis.

When we visited her at the Winston Building in January 1990, she was confined to the unit and eating from trays brought in from the cafeteria. She had been put on the old neuroleptic drug Thorazine and on Inderal for high blood pressure. She looked pale and unhappy, and she didn't understand why she couldn't go out to eat with us. When her tray came, it was anything but appetizing—cold broiled chicken (she hates chicken), cold green beans, cold boiled potatoes, a blob of fruit Jell-O, and a carton of skim milk.

At that time, in addition to her mental illness, she had sometimes fluctuating high blood pressure, high cholesterol, the kidney abnormality, and borderline anemia. Before the visit ended, Lucy cried. I was overwhelmed by the stark hospital setting, the sight of physically disabled patients sitting or lying in wheelchairs, and the now uncertain condition of Lucy's physical as well as mental health. I cried too.

In February 1990, we were told that Lucy was operating on about 15 percent of her kidney function, that by the time the lab work reflected any abnormality, 75 percent of the kidney function was already gone. We were never told exactly what caused her kidney problem, but I think it was the high doses of Tegretol and Lithium, the antipsychotic drugs that she was on at the time. In August of that year, her doctor told us that lab work showed the kidney damage wasn't as bad as first thought, and in January of 1991, he said, "Lucy can live a long time with this much kidney function."

Lucy came home for a good visit in May 1990 and seemed much improved, but she had developed a new habit of squinting her eyes. She told me she did it because "I have trouble with voices." At that time she was still very delusional and seemed to hear voices almost constantly.

The decade of the 1990s was stressful for us from beginning to end. Frank took early retirement from Tennessee Tech University in 1990 because of multiple problems relating to his diabetes. Mark's problems with manic-depression continued: he too suffered from high blood pressure and from occasional suicidal depression. He got jobs and quit jobs, overdosed on his medicine, and was hospitalized in Cookeville and at Moccasin Bend Mental Health Institute in Chattanooga.

Lucy came home for Thanksgiving 1990 and was in good spirits when we arrived at the Winston Building to pick her up. Before we left, I told one of the staff members how sorry I felt for a patient who was then confined to the unit.

She replied, "I'm sorry for all of them, and this may sound horrible, but I'd rather be dead than be in this place. There's no privacy, they have no life, they're told what to do—everything is controlled by other people. There's no individual care. If someone is doing better and might want to do more for themselves, it's always spoiled by another patient who's worse off..."

This black litany of hospital conditions was exactly what I thought, but I was shocked to hear a staff member voice it. I knew we couldn't care for Lucy at home, but I felt guilty, guilty, guilty once more.

In July 1991, I noticed Lucy's face seemed extremely sunburned and later learned that one of the drugs she was taking, Thorazine, causes sensitivity to the sun. Her face became a dark mask as the months went by, but the drug was responsible for what stability she had, and nobody mentioned changing the medication. In March 1993, Lucy's social worker called to tell me they were going to try Lucy on a new drug, Clozaril. (NOTE: Clozapine or Clozaril, which came out in the United States in 1990, can decrease white blood cells in some patients, a condition called Agranulocytosis, which can be fatal. Weekly blood counts are necessary and have to be continued every two weeks indefinitely. It can also cause cardiac problems, excessive salivation, weight gain, and sometimes diabetes.)

We were told that Lucy would be gradually taken off Thorazine, but they weren't sure her facial discoloration would go away. I was horrified to think that the condition might be permanent. Her face was still dark when she came home for visits that summer, but she was clearly better on Clozaril. Her smile no longer seemed fake, she was not responding to voices as much, and her conversation was more natural. The skin condition gradually went away. The staff on Unit A thought she was ready for discharge to a group home.

Many patients were being discharged from the hospital during the early and mid-nineties, and there was talk of closing the Winston Building again, though no money had been spent to prepare places in the community for the patients there. Frank and I visited several homes in Chattanooga during this time and thought none of them was suitable for Lucy or for anyone else.

In July 1994, Lucy was cleared for discharge to Rosewood Manor, a home for women in downtown Chattanooga. We had seen the home, an old, two-story house that was being remodeled, and thought it would be homey and so much better than the hospital. Lucy was excited about plans to leave Winston Building; she had been at the state hospital almost ten years. Finally, on October 6, 1994, Lucy called us to say she was moving to Rosewood the next day. She added, "Would you please pray I'll never have to go back to that place (Winston Building)?"

One year later, on October 2, 1995, I learned Lucy was back at Winston Building. Her doctor outside the hospital had taken her off Clozaril because he said it was not working. She was put on Clozaril again while at Winston Building and went back to Rosewood the next month. However, in February 1996, she had to be taken off the drug again because it had lowered her white blood cell count.

In March 1996, Lucy was once again hospitalized at Winston Building. When Frank and I saw her on March 14, she was pale, tearful, confused, and obviously very ill. When we saw her on March 22, her thirty-fifth birthday, she was extremely delusional and unable to go out to eat or to celebrate her birthday in any way

We picked Lucy up at the hospital on April 26 and went to Hamilton Place Mall for lunch. She was better, back on Clozaril, and had decided she wanted to live in the hospital forever—that she did not want to go back to Rosewood. We had concluded by then that Rosewood wasn't the right place for her, and we picked up her things there on May 3.

We learned that a new group home would be opened in Cowan, Tennessee, a small town west of Chattanooga; and on July 8, 1996, we met Lucy and her case manager at the Grundy County Mental Health Center in Tracy City, Tennessee, and filled out paperwork for her to stay at Cowan. The group home, located on a quiet street, was a new-looking ranch house, which had originally been built for people with mental retardation. It was nicely furnished, beautiful, and clean, and it had been newly decorated. Each client had a separate room with a big closet, and the staff members we met were professional and enthusiastic about Lucy's acceptance there. It seemed perfect, and I felt more real hope and happiness than I had in months.

Lucy's first year at Cowan went well. She came home regularly for visits and spent Thanksgiving and Christmas at home. Lucy spent her thirty-sixth birthday at home in March 1997, and although she still had problems with voices, we thought things were going well. We made the long drive to Cowan every month to pick Lucy up, ate lunch at Shoney's Restaurant in McMinnville, which she always enjoyed, and drove her back after a few days at home. The year passed without any major problems, but the spring of 1998 brought unexpected and extended trauma for Lucy.

SPRING 1998 – SPRING 2005

After spending ten years in a state mental hospital and two and a half years in group homes, Lucy was hospitalized with two potentially fatal reactions to the drugs she had been taking for twenty years.

I knew the side effects of most of the drugs she had been on: lethargy, dizziness, blurred vision, weight gain, tremors, stiffness, photosensitivity, dry mouth, nausea, and constipation were common. I knew that the older drugs could all cause Tardive Dyskinesia or TD, a serious side effect that causes movements of the tongue and mouth and sometimes movements of the arms and legs or whole body. When Lucy first went to Winston Building, I saw patients in the hospital with these grotesque, involuntary movements of mouth and limbs.

Neuroleptic Malignant Syndrome (NMS) was a more sinister side effect that I had learned of only by accident after years of dealing with schizophrenia. Many people who take antipsychotic drugs are unaware of its existence. According to information on their Web site, the National Institute of Neurological Disorders and Stroke says: "Neuroleptic Malignant Syndrome (NMS) is a life-threatening, neurological disorder most often caused by an adverse reaction to neuroleptic or antipsychotic drugs. Symptoms include high fever, sweating, unstable blood pressure, stupor, muscular rigidity, and autonomic dysfunction. In most cases, the disorder develops within the first two weeks of treatment with the drug;

however, the disorder may develop any time during the therapy period...Generally, intensive care is needed...Early identification of and treatment for individuals with neuroleptic malignant syndrome improves outcome."

On Monday, March 30, 1998, I received a phone call from a staff member at Cowan Group Home telling me that Lucy was being taken to Harton Regional Medical Center in Tullahoma, Tennessee, for evaluation and a possible medication change.

When I talked to Lucy later at the hospital, she sounded good and said, "This hospital is just like St. Thomas," referring to the hospital in Nashville where she had spent a week in June 1981. I felt better after talking with her, and Frank and I planned to see her the following Tuesday.

On April 5, I spoke with a nurse in the psychiatric unit at Harton who told me that Lucy was better and was being given Olanzapine (Zyprexa), one of the newer drugs for schizophrenia that came out in 1996. When we saw Lucy on Tuesday, April 7, we found her tired-looking and slow in speech. She was not talking to voices as much, but she said she still heard them. Lucy was discharged from Harton and returned to Cowan Group Home on April 10.

When I called the group home on April 11, a staff member told me Lucy was not doing well—that she couldn't sit still, was sweating heavily, and her blood pressure was abnormal—symptoms I now believe were early indicators of NMS. When I spoke to Lucy, she spoke haltingly with long silences between words. I told the staff member that she needed help, and she was taken back to

Harton Medical Center that day.

When I called Lucy at the hospital on April 12, she was hardly coherent with long gaps between her words. She told me she felt "worse and worse." Had I known then what I know now, I would have left for the hospital immediately, but because I spoke with staff and with her doctor frequently, I felt she was being monitored closely and there was no cause for alarm.

On Friday morning, April 17, Frank and I drove to Harton hospital expecting to find Lucy better. I remember punching the button to be let into the psychiatric unit, and someone then directing us to her room. We found her sitting on the side of her bed in a crouched position with her arms held out in front of her in a stiff, fixed posture. There was a yellowish coloration under her eyes, which were bloodshot and unblinking. I touched her face and found it cold and clammy. She seemed to be paralyzed and in a catatonic state. I didn't know if she knew us, but I felt strongly that she wanted to speak and couldn't.

The shock and horror of finding her unattended in that condition has blurred my memory of the rest of that morning as we frantically tried to find out what had happened to her and what could be done. I remember thinking of NMS but it was not then confirmed. At my request, the staff moved her to a room with a hospital bed, and she was subsequently put on IVs. Her doctor had called in a neurologist, but he didn't arrive until 2 p.m. Those hours of waiting were agonizing, and I couldn't hold back tears whenever I looked at Lucy, who remained in a rigid, catatonic state.

NMS was confirmed when the neurologist finally arrived. He told us Lucy's vital signs, renal function, and temperature were all right, and he put her on a drug that he said would make the rigidity go away in a day or two.

The rigidity disappeared, but in the following weeks we found Lucy incontinent, eating little, delusional at times, and slow in speech with no expression in her face. On April 22, a friend from Cookeville drove with me to see Lucy. The stench of urine greeted us before we entered her room at the end of a hall. We found Lucy lying in a wet bed in soiled clothes with matted, dirty hair, clearly unaware of her condition. She was very thirsty, and I got her two containers of orange juice from a snack bar on the unit, which she gulped down. I went to the nurses' station and told them what I thought about the lack of care she was getting when she obviously could not take care of herself. My anger at the situation has blotted out my exact words, but nobody contradicted me, and a student nurse got clean towels and helped Lucy down to the showers.

Two cleaning women came back to the unit to change her bed again. One of them told me that she had seen Lucy wet herself before they left the unit earlier, but didn't tell anyone because she thought the nursing staff would take care of it. I wondered how long she might have stayed that way if we hadn't come. I was especially concerned that she needed help eating and drinking and apparently had not been getting it.

Her doctor talked with us very sympathetically, and I felt that he was doing everything he could to help her recover. When I called the hospital on April 24, the nurse told me Lucy was getting psychotic (she had been taken off all the neuroleptic drugs), wasn't eating much, was very restless at night, and was "not doing well at all." During the night a staff member had found her standing up on her bed, jumping up and down.

Frank and I went to Tullahoma the next day, and I wrote this after the visit: "haunted by Lucy as we found her yesterday—troubled looking, delusional, hardly seemed to know what she was doing...Beautiful weather makes me sad when I think of all the springs she's spent locked up, unable to enjoy anything because of this hellish illness."

On May 12, the hospital called to tell us that Lucy was running a fever, her white cell count had suddenly dropped, and she was being moved to a MedSurg unit.

Frank and I drove to Tullahoma the next morning, and I planned to stay in the Hampton Inn across from the hospital until Lucy was better. We found her pale and nauseated, and after Frank left, I stayed with her until 7 p.m. She had received good treatment and seemed much better when I saw her the next morning, May 14. She was more lucid, relaxed, in good spirits, and seemed better than I had seen her in many months. Throughout the day, she talked, smiled, and seemed glad of my presence. It was a happy respite that I later wrote about as follows:

RESPITE

I sit by her hospital bed,

Silently rejoicing at the lucid smile
In her soft, blue eyes.
Close, touching, laughing,
United by memories,
Shared years, endless tears,
The baby girl
I bore so long ago.
Now, thirty-seven,
Her young, best days
Spent locked away,
Endless hospitalizations,
Drugs, demons, doctors,
Frantic fears,
Hollow dreams,
Cackling voices,
Waiting to return.

The next day, Lucy was still doing well, and her doctor told me she would be transferred by ambulance to Moccasin Bend Mental Health Institute that morning. I had hoped she might go back to Cowan, but was glad she would be taken by ambulance. I called home and told Frank I would probably be ready to leave the hospital by noon. When he and Mark arrived, Lucy was still waiting, and we had learned nothing about when she would leave.

We went out for lunch, came back and then began a nightmare day of uncertainty and waiting. At mid-afternoon, I learned no ambulance had been called because TennCare (Tennessee's medical insurance for the poor, uninsured, and disabled) had not cleared it. I went to the administrator's office in tears of frustration, but was told they could do nothing. As the hours dragged on, Lucy began deteriorating, and I was acutely aware of Frank and Mark waiting to leave, not understanding the endless delay. Finally, around 5 p.m., we had to leave, unsure of how or when she would be transported to Moccasin Bend. When I left, she was growing delusional and had started taking her clothes off, putting on her nightgown, clearly regressing. I felt totally thwarted by the system once more.

When we got back to Cookeville after 6 p.m., I called the hospital and learned that she was still waiting. I was finally told that she had been taken to Moccasin Bend by two police officers after the TennCare driver refused to make the trip because he thought she was going back to Cowan. The nurse told me that she was glad that the TennCare driver didn't take Lucy after she got a look at him, which added to my anxieties about the kind of people TennCare hired to transport patients. I later learned that Lucy was given a bed at Moccasin Bend around 11 that night.

Lucy's recovery from NMS at Moccasin Bend stretched from May until September 1998 and became for me a period of continuing stress and shock as we tried to follow her treatment. Mark and I visited her on May 17, and I was told by a psychiatric tech that Lucy was better than the day before when "she was running up and down the halls—just *flying.*" Lucy came out to the visiting area accompanied by a technician and smiled and seemed glad to see us. She had just had a bath, and her hair was wet, so I asked for a towel and dried and combed her hair while we were there. She was pale, with dry lips and a blank expression, and she seemed extremely tired. She suddenly said, "I'm going back to bed," and we had to buzz for someone to let her into the unit again.

On May 22, I drove to the hospital alone for a meeting with her psychiatrist and other "team" members. I was met on her unit by the hospital's patient advocate who told me Lucy had been "hurting herself," that she had a black eye, had been "banging into things," and had fallen out of a chair, news that filled me with apprehension. I had to sign some papers and then met with her psychiatrist, nurses, and others involved. Her doctor at that meeting seemed very understanding and interested in all the history I could relate about Lucy's past and present condition. I signed permission papers for him to try her on one of the newer antipsychotic drugs, Risperidone (Risperdal). Anything seemed better than her present condition.

Before the meeting ended, Lucy was brought into the room. She was dressed in a blue smock and had a huge black eye, dark bruises on both arms, and was totally incoherent, though she did recognize me. I hugged her and asked what had happened to her eye. She replied, "I popped it out." She was not able to sit still and was taken back to her room. I made plans to meet with the doctor and staff weekly and, though I was stunned by her appearance, I felt, at that time, that she was in good hands.

I called the hospital regularly and was told that Lucy was still incontinent, was not eating much, and had to be restrained in a geriatric or "gerry chair" to keep her from falling. When I spoke with her doctor on May 27, I learned she was still "hurting herself" but was "not quite as frightened," and he thought she was not as bad as when I saw her five days earlier. He also told me his wife was expecting a baby at any time and that he might not be available when I came down again.

I was already obsessed by Lucy's condition, and when Frank and I went to Chattanooga on May 28, a staff member rolled her out in a gerry chair, wearing diapers and pajamas that were obviously too tight. Her hair and ears were dirty, and she had two black eyes with blood spots in them and extensive bruising around her neck and along her hairline. She looked at us briefly but mostly stared ahead and held her mouth open and rigid for periods. Her doctor was available, and I felt better after talking with him and showing him the bruising, though he gave me no satisfactory reason for it. He said she was being given liquids and that she was tolerating the Risperdal. I couldn't understand how she could have blackened her eyes and bruised herself so badly when she was supposed to be closely monitored, but the only explanation I was given was that she had "hurt herself."

The next day, Friday, May 29, I got a call from the hospital a little before 8 p.m. telling me that Lucy had had a series of seizures, "one after another," and had been taken to Erlanger Hospital. Frank and I decided to drive to Erlanger the next morning, and I spent a good part of Friday night calling the hospital, only to get sketchy information about her condition. She arrived unconscious and was on a ventilator in the ICU, but her condition was stable when I made a last call around midnight.

The next morning we took our little Chihuahua, Moody, to the veterinarian's and drove the 100 miles to Chattanooga, filled with dread once more. The town was crawling with tourists and unfamiliar traffic, but we finally found the hospital and saw Lucy around noon. She was in the ICU, in four-point restraints, a ventilator tube down her throat, on IVs, fear and misery reflected in her bloodshot eyes. Her mouth was badly bruised, and she was constantly trying to move her arms and legs and flex her body. It was like watching an animal tied down. I don't think I ever saw her in worse condition, but her nurse said they might take the ventilator out later after some tests.

All the downtown hotels were filled, but the hospital helped us get a room in one of them through some arrangement they had, and we thankfully checked in. The next day I called the hospital early and was told that Lucy had been restless but had not been extremely agitated during the night. The ventilator was out, and she had been drinking grape juice and did not seem unhappy; she was singing a Neil Diamond song that was playing on the unit at one point.

We saw her after breakfast, and I was so thankful the ventilator tube was gone. She was still thrashing her legs and arms and her breathing was noisy; her throat was probably sore from the ventilator. The doctor who treated her there asked me about the bruises she still had around her face and neck and on her arms and legs, some of which were old. I told him the staff at Moccasin Bend had told me "she did it herself."

Lucy received excellent care at Erlanger for the four days she was there, and she was discharged June 2 and returned to her unit at Moccasin Bend. I never received any satisfactory answer for the extensive bruising she showed on that unit and contacted the Tennessee Protection and Advocacy Agency for help in determining what had happened. One of their advocates met me at Moccasin Bend on June 5 and helped me in talking with staff and getting Lucy transferred to another unit where she remained until discharge on September 23, 1998.

As a family member, I remember little sympathetic treatment from the staff on her previous unit—none from the second doctor who treated her there—and no satisfactory answer to any of my questions about her condition. I had an investigation made by the state hospital's investigator about possible abuse, but nothing could be proved. I know it's possible Lucy did injure herself, but at no time do I recall a staff person from that unit ever sitting down to talk with me about how that had happened. I am left with the impression that, at the least, she was neglected there.

My memory of that whole period is colored by my own stress and grief at her condition, but I have a clear memory of the unit she was moved to. I recall walking in and seeing the charge nurse standing with her arm around a patient, listening to her concerns. She only spoke to me when she had finished her conversation with this patient, and I was mightily impressed by this caring attitude. Also, I remember that the doctor, nurses, and other staff there readily gave me information about Lucy's condition when I met with them. This kind of consideration means so much to family members, and I think anyone who works in a hospital, especially a mental hospital where patients may not be able to voice their concerns clearly, should be aware of how far small kindnesses go to relieve stress.

Lucy's recovery extended from weeks to months with little improvement to celebrate when we visited her. She remained incontinent, was not eating normally, and was usually incoherent or totally silent, sometimes gesturing with her arms, sometimes staring blankly ahead with no response to our attempts at conversation. Had it not been for her doctor's patience in trying different drugs and combinations of drugs, his optimism that she would get better, and the nursing care she got from the staff then, I couldn't have made it through a single visit without breaking down. I started seeing a therapist in Cookeville in July and also got a prescription for an antidepressant for the crushing depression that had settled over me like a wet, smothering blanket.

In late August Lucy became very psychotic again. She was screaming and yelling when I called the unit, but she seemed more herself when Frank and I saw her a few days later. She gave both of us big hugs and was enthusiastic about a diet Pepsi I brought her from the snack bar. Then she suddenly remarked, "Please don't come to visit me again—ever." Her dinner tray was brought in and placed on a table in the visiting area, but she picked it up and went back inside to eat. We could see her talking to voices in the dining area, and the visit ended.

Finally, on September 23, when she had been tried on a combination of Clozaril and Zyprexa, real improvement began, and she returned to Cowan Group Home. She was doing better than we had seen her in years, physically and mentally, when she came home for a visit in October 1998. That's when we had the portrait made that appears on the cover of this book.

Her white blood count was then in the "low normal" range, but in November, it had dropped below normal, and she had to be taken off Clozaril again. She had a good leave home for Christmas that year, but in February 1999, she was taken to Greer House, a halfway home just outside of Moccasin Bend Mental Health Institute, for evaluation and a possible med change. She has never been able to tolerate Clozaril again, and she has never been as well as for the brief period in 1998 after recovering from NMS.

Weight gain became a major problem over the years, partly caused by Zyprexa and other drugs. She was hospitalized five or six times between May 1999 and February 2000. She was able to come home for Thanksgiving and Christmas in 1999, but the effect of all these hospitalizations was unending stress for us as we traveled to the different hospitals, met with whatever doctor was treating her, and tried to find some hope when different drugs were tried. Nothing seemed to work for long. Every hospitalization took its toll on Lucy in confusion and readjustment, and I continued to be amazed at her resilience.

Anyone not familiar with serious mental illness may wonder what caused the repeated hospitalizations. When Lucy has been with us for visits home or just out to eat either from the hospital or a group home, I've never seen her completely free of the symptoms of her illness: hearing voices, inability to concentrate for long periods, and disordered thoughts. At her best, she's always been aware of her surroundings, has never at her sickest failed to recognize her family, and is usually cheerful and affectionate and able to enjoy going for a drive, eating a good meal, listening to a favorite Billy Joel or James Taylor song, and other simple pleasures.

Signs that she is not doing well include the inability to sleep, either eating enormous amounts of food or not eating at all, and increasing distraction by voices that finally make it impossible for her to do anything at all. I have seen and heard her at home in her room, sweating heavily, screaming and shouting responses to the devilish voices she's never been free of since this illness took over. Sometimes she speaks in harsh, guttural tones and sometimes in a whining, little-girl voice. When this behavior continues over days without respite, this means another hospitalization and more drug trials. The process is unnerving and confusing for Lucy and stressful for those who love her.

I know that Lucy may never be completely free of the voices and the delusional thinking. I believe God hears her prayers and understands her often unintelligible words, but I no longer try to make sense of some of the things she says. These are fragments of her conversation I copied recently: "I'm sorry I didn't wash my face but there was a boy who had a gun but luckily I turned the gun into a bag of winter-fresh mints and saved his life…" "I thought I was all right, a nice young woman, but then he had another test and I had to become a born-again-Christian to get out of the Slough of Despond…"

After her hospitalization at Moccasin Bend in February 2000, we were told that she would not be able to go back to Cowan Group Home. After anxious days wondering where she could go, we were told she was eligible for a home in Pikeville, Tennessee, which was only sixty-five miles from Cookeville. We visited the home and were elated that she would be this close to home and in such a good place.

On March 17, 2000, Lucy went to Brookview Group Home and sounded very happy to be there when she called us later. Her time at Brookview went by so fast, looking back, and while she had some very good days there, she was hospitalized again at Moccasin Bend on April 28, 2000. Her blood pressure was high at that time, and her weight had ballooned to nearly 300 pounds. While at home in April 2001, she fell on our stairs and broke a small bone in her ankle. She wore a brace for months and developed cellulitis in her leg that May. When she wasn't stable enough to come home, Mark and I visited her in Pikeville.

She was again hospitalized at Moccasin Bend on September 28, 2001, and was not discharged until January 8, 2002. Lucy had a good visit home in April 2002, but on June 12, she was back at Moccasin Bend. She recovered quickly and was discharged on June 26. Throughout the summer of 2002, Lucy was unstable, and she was hospitalized once again at Moccasin Bend on September 20.

Nothing seemed to work for her there, and she was moved to the Winston Building on October 16. She was discharged to Brookview on November 20, still delusional and mentally fragile. She didn't come home at all for the holidays that year and saw us only for brief visits when we went to Pikeville. I wrote the following poem after Mark and I took her some Christmas gifts.

CHRISTMAS GIFT FOR MY DAUGHTER

I bought you cologne,
Slippers and a blouse,
But wish I could give
The phone call you never got from that boy in junior high,
The beau you never had,
The nursing career you wanted once,
All the days and years
You might have enjoyed
Without the chaos and the torment
Of the voices.
But I'll wrap cologne,
Slippers and a blouse,
Thankful for days
Your smile is still million-dollar bright,
Knowing how eagerly
You'll unwrap
These paltry offerings,
And give me

Something priceless in return:
Your words, "I love you Mom."

Lucy had almost constant problems during the new year, but she had lost a lot of weight, and I was thankful for that. That summer Mark went into a manic phase and was hospitalized at Moccasin Bend on July 3, 2003. He made a good recovery and was discharged July 25. Lucy was not stable enough to come home for the rest of the summer, and was taken to Moccasin Bend on October 28, after days of worsening symptoms and no sleep. A staff member at Brookview told me that Lucy was "worse than I've ever seen her."

Mark and I visited her regularly during the fall and winter of 2003 but saw little real improvement as drugs that had once worked were tried again. Due to worsening health, my husband is no longer able to make the long drive to Chattanooga.

In December we learned she had been put on medicine for hypothyroid disease. We often found her agitated and in tears, unable to respond to us at all. On March 17, 2004, she was sent back to the Winston Building, where it was thought by the staff she might do better because the units there were quieter than in the main building.

Lucy seemed calmer and more like herself when Mark and I saw her on March 21. Her forty-third birthday was March 22, and we brought a few gifts. One of mine was a stuffed animal (I've forgotten now what it was), but Lucy later asked me, "Why would a grown woman want a stuffed animal?" I was pleased by her question as it showed she was thinking more clearly. She came home for a visit for the first time in more than a year on June 27, but her eyes were bloodshot because she had been rubbing them in the shower with too much soap, and I was afraid to trust her to take a bath alone.

Lucy continued to improve over the weeks, but none of the drugs she was taking made much difference in her delusional behavior. She was calmer overall and able to enjoy going out for a hamburger or salad when Mark and I visited. After such a long period of total instability when even this wasn't possible, I was thankful for small gains. After a trip to Florida with my older son and grandchildren in July 2004, we stopped to see Lucy. She seemed glad to see all of us, but she didn't want to visit very long. Just before she went back into the unit, she told me, not for the first time, "I can't make it in the real world."

Sadly, for Lucy and others like her who are dealing with a chronic illness that has no cure, this is all too true. Whether she can ever live outside the hospital again is a question I can't answer. Movie stars and other influential celebrities don't hold fund-raisers for the severely and persistently mentally ill (SPMI). Many of them, who have no family support, or are in denial that they have an illness, are locked away in jails and prisons (prisons have become the new mental hospitals) or exist in sub-standard boarding homes or on the street. Schizophrenia is a brain disease, and there would be a huge outcry if people with other brain diseases like Parkinson's or Alzheimer's were treated this way.

Lucy came home for Christmas 2004 and made a poignant request of me: "Will you please pray that I'll have only one personality?" I told her then what I believe, that she has only one personality. In spite of everything she's been through, she is still basically kind, brave, cheerful, has a good sense of humor, and is a decent human being. This is the personality that always returns when she is at all functional.

Recently I waited for Lucy outside the locked door of her unit (families are no longer allowed inside) and looked through the small window at the top of the door. A young woman with dark hair and blue eyes came to the door with a wide smile and said, "I want to tell you Lucy is *much* better!" This is Ann (not her real name), who seems to be about Lucy's age and whom I have seen many times over the years. I smile at her and say, "Yes, she's going home for a visit."

"You look real nice," Ann responds. A psychiatric technician comes to the door and hands me a book to sign for Lucy's home leave, while holding Ann back from walking out the door. Now, Ann is at the glass again, and I wave to her, but something has changed. She doesn't wave back, but her hand is splayed across the small window, and she is moving it around and around in a cleaning motion.

"Are you cleaning the glass?" I ask, but her face is blank. Her eyes are distant and set, and only her hand continues to move methodically around and around. Then Lucy is coming toward the door with a paper bag of clothes and a big smile, calling, "Mom! My wonderful Mom!" She gives me a big hug when the door is opened, and I see that Ann has disappeared.

Too many patients like Ann and Lucy have disappeared behind locked doors because there is no place for them in the community—in the "real world." If I won the lottery tomorrow, I would provide a permanent place of care for Lucy within twenty-five miles of Cookeville so that when my husband and I are gone (he is 80; I am 77), she would at least be near her brothers.

Lucy's last group home in Pikeville was as close to what is needed as I've seen, but it's not a permanent residence. Lucy's place there was lost when she was hospitalized for so long. I would build a permanent home for perhaps eight patients that would have twenty-four-hour-awake staff trained to deal with whatever behavior arises as is done now in the hospital.

Most chronically ill mental patients also suffer from physical ailments, as in Lucy's case. A psychiatrist and a medical doctor would be on the staff to visit weekly, and while hospitalization might still be necessary at times, I believe it would be less frequent. Whatever the situation, patients like Lucy would be assured of a permanent place of care and refuge in the community near their families. Dr. E. Fuller Torrey writes about this "Need for Asylum" for the severely disabled and mentally ill in the fourth edition of his book *Surviving Schizophrenia, A Manual for Families, Consumers, and Providers.*

That June day in 1978 when Lucy first became ill is still as fresh in my mind as though it had happened yesterday. I never dreamed then how destructive schizophrenia was or that twenty-seven years later I would feel that care and services for its worst-off victims are fewer today than when we first visited a mental health center.

Years ago a psychiatrist who was then treating Lucy told me, "She's always going to be dependent." We were only a few years into this illness then. Lucy was young; I didn't believe him. But for her, the hellish symptoms of schizophrenia have never really abated. I know she needs permanent long-term care in a safe environment, and I wish with all my heart that I could provide that place for her near her family.

Lucy has never been homeless, been put in prison, or been forgotten in some dreary boarding home. She has been in continuous treatment since the day of her first breakdown. She has swallowed a staggering amount of drugs over the years, and she has suffered life-threatening side effects because of them. In spite of all this, she may never be well enough to live outside the hospital unless permanent places of care, similar to the hospital, are made available in the community. The most powerful country in the world still allows some victims of severe mental illness to live in the street, to be put in prisons, and to be shunned, ignored, and forgotten. *Catalyst,* (Winter 2003/Spring 2004) a quarterly newsletter published as a public service by the Treatment Advocacy Center in Arlington, Virginia, in an article titled, "Forty years of neglect: The federal role in caring for the severely mentally ill," states that "Today at least a third of the homeless and up to one quarter of those incarcerated have severe mental disorders such as schizophrenia and manic-depressive illness."

What will happen to Lucy when my husband and I are gone is the one constant worry we live with. This is true for all parents of disabled children. I hope I will live long enough to see that care for her, and for those like her, is assured.

In spite of the dismal record of care and services for the most severely mentally ill persons, I have hope that some research laboratory is now developing a drug that will cure this terrible illness—a drug that will allow Lucy and millions of others to emerge forever from their confusion and terrors.

For now, I try to take the advice that Lucy is constantly giving me, as she did earlier this year at a Burger King in Chattanooga. I had asked about a bruise I noticed on one of her hands.

She just laughed and said, "You worry about every little thing, Mom! God takes care of the world. Don't *worry!*"

I'm trying, Luce. I'm trying.

ACKNOWLEDGMENTS

For support, encouragement, and invaluable help in shaping *LUCY: The Anguish of Schizophrenia,* I'm deeply indebted to the following people: Janet Biery and members of Cookeville Creative Writers' Association, Inc. for listening to the new manuscript and for their suggestions; Jean Key, Susan Holland, Charles Denning, Margery Hargrove, and Thelma Johnson for giving their time to read, make corrections, and offer ideas to improve the book; and members of NAMI-Cookeville for being there and for understanding. For their constant love, encouragement and help, I want to thank my husband, our children, our daughter-in-law, and our grandchildren. I especially want to thank my son Frank for using his skill with computers to format the manuscript.

Many mental health professionals have played a part in Lucy's treatment over the years. There is no way I can list them all, but I would like to name a few I can't forget because of the kindness and respect they showed to Lucy and to her family at different times and places.

Moccasin Bend Mental Health Institute and Winston Building,

Chattanooga, Tennessee (1984-2005); Terry Holmes, MD, Clinical Director, MBMHI; Wanda Burdine, RN; Alice Reid, RN; Jane Gumnick, MD; Mitzie Thornton, Nurse Practitioner; Mike Stedman, LPN; Gary Moye, RN; Patrick Craven, MD; Claire Coffee, RN; Susan Hammond, RN; Nancy Rose, Social Worker; Tim Gossett, Psychiatric Technician; Roseanne Kelly, RN; Melanie McClendon, RN; Frances Robertson, MSN; Lakisha Hambrick, Psychiatric Technician; Mary Nunley, Psychiatric Technician; Won. Park, MD; and Beverly Miller, Counseling Associate. I would especially like to thank Rob Cotterman for his contribution to this book and for bringing a new era of openness, availability, and compassion to the Winston Building when he became director there in 1992.

Harton Regional Medical Center, Tullahoma, Tennessee, Spring 1998, Sandip Shukla, MD.

Plateau Mental Health Center, Cookeville, Tennessee, (1978-1984); Bob Freeman, CEO Volunteer Mental Health System (retired); Guy Zimmerman, MD, (deceased); Mary Eich, RN (retired); Betty Wells, RN (retired); Tommy King, LPN (retired); Lorraine Jackson, LPN (retired).

John Crabtree, MD, Cookeville, TN (for Mark, January 1980; for Lucy, May 1982).

I would like to thank the staff of Rosewood Manor (1994-1996), Cowan Group Home, (1996-2000), Brookview Group Home (2000-2003), and especially Jeani Lane, Angie Lee, and Greg Johnson.

Finally, I thank God, who has given me whatever soundness of body and mind, whatever strengths and talents that I possess. Without His grace, I could do nothing.

NOTES

1. 1 Cor. 12:12 (KJV)

2. Torrey, E. Fuller. *Surviving Schizophrenia: A Family Manual.* New York: Harper & Row, 1983.

3. Proverbs 18:14 (KJV)

4. Wordsworth, William. *Selected Poems.* New York: Penguin Classics, 2005.

5. Millay, Edna St. Vincent. *First Fig and Other Poems.* Mineola: Dover Publications, 2000.

ADVOCACY & RESOURCES

NOTE: The *Catalyst* is a quarterly newsletter published as a public service by the Treatment Advocacy Center, 3300 North Fairfax Drive, Suite 220, Arlington, VA 22201. 703-294-6001 (phone), 703-294-6010 (fax), info@psychlaws.org (e-mail)

For reading lists and other information about serious mental illness, see: the National Alliance for the Mentally Ill (NAMI), Colonial Place Three, 2107 Wilson Blvd., Suite 300, Arlington, VA 22201-3042. 703-524-7600 (phone), www.nami.org (e-mail)

NAMI-Tennessee, 1101 Kermit Drive, Suite 605, Nashville, TN 37217-2126. 615-361-6608 (phone), Web site namitn.nami.org

NAMI-Cookeville, P.O. Box 2915, Cookeville, TN 38501. 931-528-0086 (phone), wjk41@frontiernet.net (e-mail)

Recommended reading: *Surviving Schizophrenia, Fourth Edition, A Manual for Families, Consumers, and Providers* by E. Fuller Torrey, MD, copyright 2001

What is Needed

BY ROB COTTERMAN

In an ideal world, those with serious mental illnesses would be treated with a broad array of focused treatment alternatives provided on an as-needed basis. The spectrum of services would be comprised of medical, psychiatric, psychosocial, housing, and vocational education programs offered by a staff of professionals and paraprofessionals on an individualized basis to target each person's strengths and needs at any one time.

A necessary and required part of the service spectrum is the hospital. As with all services, the hospital should provide varying levels of help commensurate with a person's strength and needs, including acute and extended-care services, focused on symptom remission and rehabilitation.

Persons with severe and persistent mental illness may need treatment in a hospital when they are facing a crisis situation, and this treatment should be immediately available. Postponing hospitalization can worsen symptoms and render the climb back more difficult for the patient. A day hospital service would permit patients with less critical needs to receive treatment during the day but return to their homes in the evening.

Case management and Continuous Treatment Team (CTT) services through a PACT team (Program of Assertive Community Treatment) model would provide the broad array of support services to individuals in the community. Key to a successful PACT program is setting up services on a graduated levels system, providing them as patients' needs and desires indicate. Too intensive a service for someone who is relatively independent can smother and drive away a consumer. Too slight a service for someone whose symptoms are overwhelming is equivalent to a BAND-AID on a broken bone.

People with severe and persistent mental illness present broad differences in levels of functioning and are not well served by a single level of service for all persons. The PACT team should provide what a person requires to succeed and thrive in overcoming his illness, including, but not limited to: case management, mobile outreach, visits to consumers, psychiatric services, budgeting, grocery shopping, transportation, activities of daily living, housekeeping, social skills development, vocational services, nursing services, and short-term, focused therapy.

Crisis Response Teams (CRT) should provide swift intervention to individuals facing a psychiatric crisis. Key to the success of the CRT should be the exclusion of the law enforcement community in all but extreme cases. The accepted practice of utilizing police officers as an adjunct first line of intervention with the CRT equates the psychiatric crisis with criminal behavior. This is beyond inappropriate and takes a psychological toll on the person in crisis. CRT services should be closely integrated with PACT team members so that the person can be immediately provided with whatever is necessary and least restrictive to permit relief of his symptoms and the continuation of his life.

At the time of this writing, Lucy and other patients like her are in the hospital, which for now is the "least restrictive environment" available to provide them with needed services and supports. In an ideal world, a permanent group home for six to eight patients would be available in the community, and this would be Lucy's home. It would have twenty-four-hour-awake staff trained in understanding schizophrenia and in intervening at difficult moments that arise with patients. A nurse would be available during daytime hours, and a psychiatrist who had treated Lucy in the past and knew her medical history would provide psychiatric services.

Lucy and her peers at the home would have the benefit of a Day Treatment program and a van to take them on outings. Lucy might have the benefit of a "vocational experience" through a sheltered workshop. She would have access to services that in the past have been difficult to receive without endless referrals if she expressed a need for them or they were deemed appropriate by the staff.

If Lucy regressed, a crisis unit would instantly intervene to help her regain control. Hospitalization would be immediately available if she needed it long before she could spiral downward deep into illness. Most importantly, Lucy would have choice. All the persons intervening in her life (the home staff, her physician, day treatment staff, etc.) would understand that she is a human being with preferences, likes and dislikes, good days and bad days. Choice is a fundamental human right, but it's often lost to a person with mental illness.

In an ideal world, things would be so different for Lucy and others like her who are dealing every day with a thief—severe and persistent mental illness—that robs them of hours, days, months, and years of productive life.

Rob Cotterman, formerly Program Director of Sub-Acute Care at Moccasin Bend Mental Health Institute in Chattanooga, is Asst. Superintendent for Program Services at Moccasin Bend MHI. He received his bachelor's degree in psychology from Bryan College, and he holds a Master of Science in industrial/organizational psychology from the University of Tennessee at Chattanooga.

CPSIA information can be obtained at www.ICGtesting.com
Printed in the USA
LVOW05s0629240714

395532LV00001B/6/P

9 781583 852637